Prais

MW01178529

The Healthy Boomer:
*A No-Nonsense Midlife Health Guide for Women and Men*

"*The Healthy Boomer* provides a first-rate map of the dizzying and often distressing physical, emotional and psychological changes of midlife, providing solid help not just in surviving, but in growing as well." – *Kirkus Review*

"This book was first brought to my attention by a friend. The content is what kept me reading because it reinforces what should be obvious and often isn't – that the psychological and spiritual are as important as the physical." – Pamela Wallin, journalist

"*The Healthy Boomer* is a no-nonsense upbeat book providing easy-to-use decision-making tools, accurate information, and practical advice on health issues facing men and women in midlife." – as recommended by The North American Menopause Society

"I am convinced that all midlifers should read this boomer's bible. The writers have combined their personal and professional experience to deliver a valuable message in a refreshing, conversational tone: although midlife is a time of change, it is also a time of tremendous vitality, confidence, and joy." – Ellen Rosenberg in *Healthy Woman* magazine

"*The Healthy Boomer* will be a great source of information to help the midlife patient and doctor design a comprehensive preventive health program together. I certainly will use it with my midlife patients." – Edward Ragan, MD, private practice in Ottawa, Ontario, and specialist in public health

"Men don't go through the dramatic biological change women do, but the term male menopause has found its way into popular language – and into a new health handbook so thorough that one 53-year-old reader calls it 'my Dr. Spock for midlife.' " – Susan Schwartz, Montreal *Gazette*

"If you or your partner are one of the 10 million baby boomers in Canada facing the physical and personal challenges of midlife, *The Healthy Boomer* is a must-read." – Cheryl Embrett in *Homemakers* magazine

"*The Healthy Boomer* is a great reference tool for the health-conscious boomer, covering just about everything in a maturing adult's emotional and physical life." – Health Report, *Globe and Mail*

# THE JUGGLING ACT

## THE HEALTHY BOOMER'S
## GUIDE TO ACHIEVING BALANCE
## IN MIDLIFE

PEGGY EDWARDS,

MIROSLAVA LHOTSKY, M. D.,

AND JUDY TURNER, PH. D.

**National Library of Canada Cataloguing in Publication**

Edwards, Peggy
    The juggling act : the healthy boomer's guide to achieving balance in midlife / Peggy Edwards, Miroslava Lhotsky, Judy Turner.

ISBN 0-7710-3051-7

1. Middle aged persons – Health and hygiene.   I. Lhotsky, Miroslava
II. Turner, Judy.   III. Title

RA777.5.E383 2002      613.0434      C2002-903119-2

"If I Were a Rich Man," by Sheldon Harnick and Jerry Bock © 1964 (Renewed) Mayerling Productions Ltd. and Jerry Bock Enterprises. All rights reserved. Used by Permission Warner Brothers Publications U.S. Inc., Miami, FL 33014.

"When Death Comes" and "The Summer Day" are from *New and Selected Poems* by Mary Oliver. Copyright © 1992 by Mary Oliver. Reprinted by permission of Beacon Press, Boston.

We acknowledge the financial support of the Government of Canada through the Book Publishing Industry Development Program for our publishing activities. We further acknowledge the support of the Canada Council for the Arts and the Ontario Arts Council for our publishing program.

This book is printed on acid-free paper that is 100% ancient forest friendly (100% post-consumer recycled).

Typeset in Minion by Laura Brady
Printed and bound in Canada

McClelland & Stewart Ltd.
*The Canadian Publishers*
481 University Avenue
Toronto, Ontario
M5G 2E9
www.mcclelland.com

1 2 3 4 5    06 05 04 03 02

# CONTENTS

# Acknowledgments

There are many people who helped us develop and create this book. We are most grateful to everyone in both Canada and the United States who took the time to respond to the 2001 Healthy Boomer Midlife Survey, especially to the patients at 90 Medical Group who willingly and cheerfully answered our lengthy questionnaire. Their answers and stories were honest, reflective, and thought-provoking. We appreciate, too, that so many respondents agreed to be interviewed, even though we were unable to contact all of them. We sincerely thank these people and the experts who spoke with us in interviews. Their wisdom, openness, and experience enriched these pages enormously.

Several people helped us with the distribution and analysis of the survey questionnaire. Our thanks to:

- Harlequin Enterprises Limited, who generously made a spa gift package available to all those who completed the questionnaire, and David Galloway, former president and C.E.O. of Torstar, who kindly arranged it.
- Dr. Teresa Maryniarczyk, who kindly agreed to send questionnaires to the midlife men and women in her practice.
- Dr. Melanie MacLennan in New York, who sent our questionnaire to a sample of boomers living in the United States.
- The staff at 90 Medical, who patiently answered all questions regarding the survey and have always cheerfully taken on extra work for both *The Healthy Boomer* and this book.

- Karly Holmes, The Alder Group Inc., who supervised the input and interpretation of the data and helped us with our special requests for data analysis.

In terms of writing the book, we are indebted to:
- Suzanne Lew and Judy Field, who smooth the waters, find the information we need, and make many things possible that would not otherwise be so.
- Jo Hauser, who put up with three obsessed writers during a week of what was supposed to be a vacation, and produced excellent charts on the computer for us.
- Dr. Andrea Veisman, B.Sc., D.D.S., and Dr. Herbert Veisman, B.Sc., D.D.S., F.R.C.D.(C.), who provided expert and practical information on oral health in midlife.
- Our agent, Karen O'Reilly, who continues to encourage us and trust in us.
- Pat Kennedy, our wonderful editor at McClelland & Stewart, whose expertise and kindness vastly improve whatever crosses her desk.
- Nancy Lockhart, who has been a true friend to us and both of our books, in many important ways.

And finally, we would like to thank our families, who survived the writing of a second book and encouraged us on. We love you, Jo, Dan, Patty, Lisa, Julie, Terry, Sarah, Antonin, Lukas, and Karla.

# Introduction

Life's tragedy is that we get old too soon and wise too late.
— Benjamin Franklin, 1706–1790

## Growing Up, Growing Older

- How do you rank your health compared to that of other people your age?
- How often do you wake up feeling completely rested?
- How do you balance your work and home life?
- If there was one thing you could change in your health – physical, emotional, mental, social, or spiritual – during the coming year, what would it be?
- What is one step you can take now toward making that change?

These are some of the questions we asked some five hundred midlife women and men. Their responses were both intriguing and inspirational. They offer us something very special – heartfelt advice from our peers and the sense that we are not alone on the challenging journey of midlife.

This is a book about growing – growing up, growing older, and, we hope, growing wiser. It is about making small, incremental changes for the better in our lives and in our relationships. It is about restoring and reinventing ourselves as we strive to manage the stresses of the midlife transition.

In the pages that follow, men and women in the baby-boom generation – those born between 1946 and 1964 – talk about how they have learned to accept aging, make healthful changes, and enjoy midlife. When we asked what change they would most like to make in the next year, the answers ranged from "lose weight" and "get more exercise" to "explore the spiritual side of my life" and "spend more time with my children or grandchildren." Our conversations with boomers also shed light on how to cope

1

with things we cannot change – such as the death of a loved one, the loss of a job, or the onset of a chronic illness. Many members of the generation that vowed to be forever young and carefree have learned how important it is to thrive, not just survive, when times are tough.

We are deeply grateful to the men and women who shared their conflicted feelings about growing up and their deepest thoughts about growing older. While growing older is inevitable, many boomers are not so sure that they want to grow up. Many yearn for the fun and adventure of their youth at the same time that they enjoy the perks of adulthood. They are actively and sometimes desperately trying to find that elusive balance between work, home, and play. In the wake of two recessions and the terrorist attack of September 11, 2001, many boomers are questioning what it really means to have "the good life" they have worked so hard to achieve. They tell us again and again that family, friends, love, laughter, and simple things are the essence of joy in everyday life.

## Why We Wrote This Book

It took the three of us – a physician, a psychologist, and a health promotion consultant – more than five years to research and write our first book, *The Healthy Boomer: A No-Nonsense Midlife Health Guide for Women and Men*. We joked about birthing an elephant and calling our next book *The Haggard Boomer*. As full-time, self-employed professionals, wives, mothers, and daughters, we struggled to juggle our home and work lives. We spent would-be holidays with our computers and worked late into the night.

In between marathon writing efforts, we tried to keep our own hormone roller-coaster rides on track. Our weekly to-do lists brought on hot flashes. We cried over loved ones lost to breast cancer and AIDS, became parents and grandparents, nudged teenagers out of the nest, sea-kayaked in a mini hurricane, and took on a public-health mission in Palestine. Through it all, we struggled to follow the advice we were writing about in *The Healthy Boomer*.

After our book was published, in 1999, we embarked on a flurry of media interviews and then a series of workshops with health professionals and men and women in midlife. In a radio interview, Peggy described how one reader had called *The Healthy Boomer* her "Dr. Spock for midlife." We knew we had reached middle age ourselves when the young interviewer looked puzzled and then said, "Oh yes, isn't he the guy with the pointy ears?"

In seminars, we adopted a practical metaphor for the midlife experience, by asking people to juggle three balls. Most had little trouble throwing and catching the first ball – dubbed "work." There were a few mishaps when the second ball – dubbed "family, friends, and homelife" – was added. Bedlam broke loose when people added the third ball – aptly labeled "me."

Like us, participants found it almost impossible to juggle the responsibilities of midlife and still find time and energy for themselves. Over and over, we heard how a lack of balance keeps us stuck in the revolving door of the middle years. In discussions about personal health, one phrase was repeated over and over, "I know what I should do to stay healthy, but I just don't have the time."

We knew from our clinical work as well as our own experiences that translating the principles of good health into daily action is frustrating and difficult. While this dilemma is not unique to midlife, research increasingly shows how the personal health and lifestyle choices we make now will significantly determine how we look and feel over the next thirty years.

We also heard about the good things – how men in their fifties felt more comfortable with intimacy, and how midlife women felt freer and less afraid that people are judging them by their looks. We heard how both men and women enjoyed the sense of accomplishment and independence that comes with experience and maturity. We heard about their love of family and friends and their eagerness to give back to the community through volunteer work.

In our seminars, participants are always pleased to hear others' stories of struggle and success. For example, whenever someone tells a story about not being able to find her glasses, or her car in the parking lot, inevitably there is laughter, then sighs of relief – "Oh good, I'm not the only one." This is followed by an outpouring of other stories and strategies that leaves us all feeling heartened and not so alone.

The men and women who grew up in the boomer generation have always looked to their peers for inspiration and advice. (Ironically, we were the generation that swore to "never trust anyone over thirty.") It made sense to ask them – not only the health experts – about the best ways to manage midlife. To help us do this, we decided to conduct a midlife health survey and follow it up with personal interviews. This book is the result.

### About the Healthy Boomer Midlife Survey

The 2001 Healthy Boomer Midlife Survey used a non-random questionnaire to elicit a sense of common issues and solutions for people in midlife. We coupled this with telephone interviews to draw out some in-depth ideas on managing this period of life.

We mailed out some 500 questionnaires to almost equal numbers of men and women born between 1946 and 1964. In addition, we were pleased to receive some responses from women and men born in the decade before 1946. Considering the length of the questionnaire, the response rate was high (42 per cent). We received 210 completed questionnaires within the time limit we allowed. All of these contained a number of core questions. Then we divided the sample into three, asking one third more detailed questions about relationships, one third about work, income, retirement, spirituality, and dying, and one third about lifestyle and appearance.

The sample that received the survey was drawn largely from our professional practices in the Toronto area; some 150 questionnaires were also sent to people who live in other parts of Canada and the United States. Most of the respondents live in middle-income circumstances and have attained some level of education or training beyond high school. As expected in this kind of group, the majority are in good physical health, although some people are coping with chronic illnesses. As you will read later, the "score" on emotional well-being was more problematic. Family situations varied, from single to married, from parents of young children to grandparents. The majority are (over)employed, and some are between jobs and a few are retired. A high number of respondents are self-employed.

The majority of respondents were in their mid- to late forties and fifties. We were pleased – but not surprised – by the large response we got from men, both in sending back their completed questionnaires and in agreeing to be interviewed. Many people believe that midlife men are uninterested in health and are reluctant to talk about it. On the contrary, we have found in our previous research and in our practices that men are every bit as concerned as women about their health and the changes they are undergoing in midlife. Unfortunately, our culture does little to encourage them to talk about these concerns. But when men are asked to share their experiences with loving partners, close friends, or trusted health professionals, they are eager to do so.

We have used statistics from our survey sparingly in the book to draw attention to some common themes. At times, we compare our findings to those of larger surveys, such as the National Population Health Survey (Canada, 1996/97) and the National Survey on Midlife Development (U.S., 1995/96). However, the heart of this book lies in the anecdotes, quotes, and stories we found in the questionnaires and followup interviews. We leave it to you to determine how meaningful our findings are, compared to your own experiences in midlife.

### SOME HIGHLIGHTS FROM THE HEALTHY BOOMER MIDLIFE SURVEY

*Do you have a fulfilling sexual relationship?*

|  | Men | Women |
|---|---|---|
| Always | 17% | 11% |
| Most of the time | 50% | 36% |
| Some of the time | 28% | 42% |
| Never | 5% | 11% |

*In an average week, how many hours do you sleep each night?*

| More than 8 hours | 3% |
|---|---|
| About 8 hours | 35% |
| 5 to 7 hours | 58% |
| Less than 5 hours | 4% |

*Do you plan to retire?*

| Gradually | 48% |
|---|---|
| All at once | 19% |
| Not at all | 21% |
| No answer/undecided | 12% |

---

*Are you comfortable with your current weight?*

| | |
|---|---|
| Yes | 35% |
| No | 65% |

---

## How to Use This Book

In her poem "The Summer Day," in *New and Selected Poems* (1992), poet Mary Oliver asks:

> Tell me, what is it you plan to do
> with your one wild and precious life?

This is an important question for boomers. In midlife, we start to realize that life on earth is temporary and precious. There are so many things we want to do and so little time in our busy schedules to do them.

In this book, each chapter provides you with various ways you might answer Oliver's question. There are motivating ideas and stories from boomers you know and don't know, brief updates from the scientific literature that have come to light since *The Healthy Boomer* was published in 1999, and some interesting findings from the 2001 Healthy Boomer Midlife Survey. In most chapters, we have included a section called "On the Lighter Side." We have received these stories and quotes over the past five years from readers and friends, usually via e-mail. They brightened our days and helped us put midlife in perspective. We hope they will do the same for you.

You do not need to read each chapter in sequence; you can go immediately to a subject that is currently on your mind. We do suggest, however, that you read Chapter 2 – "Shifting Focus: Making Changes That Last." It provides a theoretical but practical approach for understanding personal change that will help you carry through on changes that you want to make and that are discussed in the other chapters. Each chapter ends with some questions on which to reflect. We hope they will inspire you to take that first, second, or third step toward taking charge of your health now.

# CHAPTER ONE

# So You Think You're Healthy, Eh?: Emotional Health in Midlife

Beaver: Gee, there's something wrong with just about everything, isn't there, Dad?
Ward: Just about, Beav.
   – Father and son talk in *Leave It to Beaver* (1957–1963)

Remember the long-running television show *Leave It to Beaver* and the perfect suburban life it showed? Even in this 1950s, sugary, made-for-television sitcom, the Beav knew there was something wrong. For the boomers who participated in our survey, the something that is wrong has far more to do with our psychological well-being than with our physical health. Depression, anxiety, insomnia, fear of memory loss, and other emotional problems are part of how we define the totality of what we call our health. It is time we talked about it.

One of the most revealing findings of the 2001 Healthy Boomer Midlife Survey was the discrepancy between how people perceived their health – which most of us think of in physical terms only – and what they told us about their emotional well-being. More than 82 per cent of respondents said that their health was "excellent," "very good," or "good." At the same time, 67 per cent said they suffered from anxiety, depression, or occasionally depressed feelings. A full one-third was also dealing with insomnia. Many expressed the fear of losing their memories.

In addition, when we asked people to identify the one thing they would like to change in the next year, half gave answers related to emotional well-being. Our midlife participants wanted to worry less, relax more, and find a better balance between work, play, and rest.

In this chapter we explore how boomers are dealing with emotional and mental-health issues in midlife.

## Trouble in Paradise?

So what is going on? Why is there so much distress in the paradise we boomers have worked so hard to achieve? And why do we still tend to think of health as physical only, despite our generation's interest in the holistic concept of an integrated mind, body, and spirit?

Part of the problem may be that we have a health-care system that focuses on (and pays for the treatment of) physical problems far more often than emotional and mental difficulties. Another part might be our underlying reluctance to admit that we suffer from emotional distress. How often have you said to yourself, "Just pull up your socks, and these feelings will go away"? Too often we judge emotional distress as a sign of weakness or a character flaw.

The World Health Organization predicts that in twenty years depression will be the world's number-one public-health problem. Last year in Canada, almost fourteen million prescriptions for antidepressants were filled. This figure attests to the prevalence of depression in our society and to the discrepancy between how we say we feel and how we really are. We hope that, at least to some extent, it also represents our greater willingness to seek help and the increased effectiveness of some of the new drugs we have for treating a wide range of mental-health problems.

### SOME HIGHLIGHTS FROM THE HEALTHY BOOMER MIDLIFE SURVEY

| *How do you rate your health compared to that of other people your age?* | |
| --- | --- |
| Excellent | 21% |
| Very good | 31% |
| Good | 31% |
| Fair | 10% |
| Poor | 2% |
| No answer | 5% |

| *Do you have health problems that interfere with your day-to-day functioning?* | |
| --- | --- |
| No | 64% |
| Yes | 26% |

| *Have you experienced in the last ten years or are you now experiencing (more than one answer is possible) . . . ?* | |
|---|---|
| Panic attacks | 14% |
| Anxiety | 20% |
| Occasional depression | 46% |
| Depression | 22% |
| Insomnia | 33% |
| Other emotional-health concerns | 4% |
| None of above | 13% |

### What's Wrong with Me?

It is normal for people of all ages to feel depressed or suffer anxious moods from time to time. Boomers in our survey were most likely to describe these feelings in two ways: as a pervasive sense of feeling overwhelmed and as a longing for joy that they seem to have lost somehow. A lack of capacity for pleasure is one of the complaints we hear most often in our clinic and our practices. When fatigue and exhaustion are added, many people worry that they are "going crazy." They need reassurance that this is not the case.

One person said, "I feel withdrawn and exhausted; I don't want to do anything." Another said, "Feeling depressed makes it very difficult to cope with daily life and everything becomes a struggle." A depressed mood and exhaustion are often coupled with an inability to focus. Respondents spoke of having difficulty concentrating and of feeling unmotivated and distracted. One man said he could not trust his own judgment and his ability to make decisions when he was feeling this way.

Many people pointed out that symptoms of depression and anxiety affected their relationships and made communication difficult. They spoke about being crabby, impatient, and short-tempered on the one hand, and withdrawn and uncommunicative on the other hand. "My exhaustion affects my marriage and my relationships with my children, and forces me to 'perform' at work," said one woman (who coincidentally ranked her health as "very good").

Irritability, anxiety, and feeling down were key factors that midlife women and men most wanted to change in the coming year. "Worry" was a consistent theme. One woman said, "Worrying seems to be hereditary or at least learned in childhood. I have to stop worrying about what other people think."

Our survey was conducted before the terrorist attacks of September 11, 2001, that so dramatically altered the sense of security most boomers have always taken for granted. Many note heightened anxiety and feelings of helplessness in the face of this event over which we had no control. There is no easy answer to the complexity of feelings aroused, but Niebuhr's Serenity Prayer that Alcoholics Anonymous uses points us in the right direction. We must somehow learn to have "the courage to change the things we can, the patience to accept the things we can't change, and the wisdom to know the difference."

In our survey, men and women were almost equally likely to report depressed or anxious feelings, although Canadian statistics suggest that, in the middle years, women are twice as likely to report depression. In our clinics, we hear many men say, "I am not depressed; I'm just tired." It seems to be harder for them to admit to depression than it is for women. Unfortunately, our culture still idealizes the macho "I'll stick it out" attitude for men and sanctions the use of alcohol as a defence against feeling too much. Boomer men often distance themselves in close relationships for the same reason.

Both men and women were more conscious of their own moodiness than that of their partners. More than one-third of men admitted to "grumpiness and sadness," and almost half to feeling "a lack of energy." Women noted these feelings in their male partners about 25 per cent of the time. Interestingly, the men were more in tune with the women than cultural norms would suggest. Almost half said their female partners suffered mood swings. This was exactly the same percentage of women in the menopausal period who said the same. "Mood swings and feeling anxious are what I find most difficult," said one woman. "There are days that I feel hateful; then the next day my reactions are totally different. Sometimes I feel sad, and I cry for no apparent reason."

There are significant differences between "feeling down" and having a major depressive episode. It is useful to think about depressed feelings on a continuum. These range from mild and transitory feelings – a blue day – to the more chronic dysthymia, the common cold of depressive feelings.

With dysthymia, people are often very self-critical, negative, and pessimistic, but continue to function. From here, the continuum moves to the major depressive episode, which is acute and debilitating. At this end of the continuum, people are unable to function in basic tasks.

As with any condition of unwellness, it is important not to isolate yourself and not to self-medicate. If milder symptoms persist for more than two weeks and/or you have acute depressive feelings that include thoughts of suicide, see your family physician right away.

**James** told us that he had suffered from mild depression for a long time before he decided to go for help. "It went on for quite a few years. I was not sociable at all, and I used to think, 'Well, I guess I am just in a bad mood.' But the bad mood continued for a very long time! Finally I went to my physician. It helped that I have known him for many years and consider him a friend, but it was still very hard – kind of like going to 'confession.' When I started on the medication, it reminded me of what it was like when I was about fifteen years old and went to be fitted for glasses for the first time. When you put those glasses on, you suddenly see what you have been missing! I had forgotten how good one can feel and how well one can function when you aren't always feeling angry and obsessive about small things."

James was able to share his experience with one of his best friends and with family members. "I had to tell my son," he said, "to explain some of my behavior towards him and why I used to overreact. Once I told him, I think he understood, and I felt better. I realized that my father suffered from depression as well, and I talked to him about it. He finally admitted that he was depressed. He said, 'I am sorry, because if it is hereditary you got it from me.'"

What advice does James give to other boomers who may be depressed but are afraid or hesitant to seek help? "I would tell them about my experience and how it worked for me," he says. "I would tell them to pay more attention. It happens so gradually that you may not be aware of how depressed you are until you go for help."

For midlife men and women going through major depressive episodes, the symptoms can be overwhelming. Said another man, "My sense of resilience and hope has been eroded. I have experienced a tremendous sense of loss, a weakened spirit and body. A sense that my life is so very small." Yet another person spoke about the loss of self-esteem that often accompanies mental and emotional distress. "I feel stripped of my spirit and good feelings," she said. "I have lost my self-esteem and self-confidence about who I really am."

Fortunately, more people are talking openly now about their struggles with depression, including a number of well-known celebrities, such as actor Margot Kidder and ex-Olympic athlete Elizabeth Manley. Even the angst-ridden boomer icon Leonard Cohen seems no longer to be wracked with bouts of depression. Cohen spent six years at the highly disciplined Mount Baldy Zen Monastery doing strenuous physical labor, coupled with an intense program of silent meditation. He emerged from this lengthy retreat to record a new album and even consider a concert tour. In an interview with the Toronto *Globe and Mail* in September 2001, he said, "I have certainly battled depression over the years and my time on Mount Baldy was one of the remedies. I liked the life there . . . it's not an easy life but it's a simple one."

### Sorry, What Did You Say Your Name Is Again?

Memory lapses in midlife cause boomers great distress. Many worry that they are "losing their grip" and that Alzheimer disease is only one forgotten name away. A professional woman in her early fifties put it this way: "I have become used to running up the stairs, only to have to run back down, hoping I will then remember what I went up for in the first place! I try to comfort myself by saying, 'Oh well, I get a little more exercise that way.'"

Another boomer said, "What really unnerved me was running into a colleague and drawing a complete blank in place of her name. Where did it go? I took a deep breath. I have learned that if I don't panic, the name will come back to me sooner."

Louise Plouffe, a psychologist and specialist in aging who works with the Division of Aging and Seniors at Health Canada, explains that memory declines typically do not show up in standardized performance tests until much later than midlife. "Normally, there is no noticeable difference in memory skills until after age seventy," she says. "Forgetfulness in midlife is more likely due to other factors, such as information overload and the stress of balancing work and family, than it is to a change in brain functioning. Women who aren't sleeping well due to hot flashes in menopause may find it hard to concentrate during the day, and feel that they are losing their memory. People in their forties and fifties also tend to be more aware that they are aging than adults in their thirties. We notice our wrinkles and may feel a touch of arthritis. So we begin to attend more to our memory and think we are forgetting more. In reality, with how busy people are in midlife, I am amazed at how much we do remember!"

Should we fear encroaching Alzheimer disease when we find ourselves forgetting? "The number of cases of Alzheimer disease under the age of sixty-five is extremely small," Louise says. "If someone really is experiencing memory loss in midlife, I would be more concerned about the relationships between forgetfulness and stress, depression, or a Vitamin B deficiency, rather than Alzheimer disease."

**Strategies for Change**

Boomers talked about what they perceived as the major barriers to changing the state of their emotional health. These included a need to work long hours to make enough money (and the fatigue and irritability that result from this), unresolved conflicts from the past, cultural differences between generations, perfectionism, a need for control (which makes them unable to let go of any responsibilities), and the lack of a cooperative partner.

The boomers in our survey suggested a number of strategies for dealing with memory mishaps. "We need to keep things in perspective," said one woman. "When all is said and done, I rarely forget the things that are really important." Others talked about maintaining a sense of humor and laughing about "forgetfulness boo-boos."

"Reducing stress and overload is a key strategy," says Louise Plouffe. "When we are anxious and stressed, it is easy to get distracted and forget things. There are also some specific tricks for improving memory, such as repeating a name when you first hear it and making a link in your mind that will help you remember it. For example, I was just introduced to a new colleague at work who has the same name as my niece. Once I made that association, I knew I would remember her name. Writing things down is also a key strategy. Even if you forget your grocery list, the fact that you have written down the items you need will help you remember them as you go up and down the aisles."

Several people in our survey said that their memories seemed to improve when they took on new jobs and learned new things. Louise Plouffe explains the biology behind this observation. "As adults, we create some new 'nodes' of information in the brain like children do, but more importantly we create new linkages among things we already know, but hadn't associated before. We see more possibilities and more layers of meaning than ever before. Probably the most important factors at work in the situation of a new job or new learning, however, are novelty – we are biologically wired to attend to novelty and to tune out familiarity – and personal motivation. Both of these enhance learning at any age. We become more alert and more attentive. In my own experience, I come alive when I attend my personal-interest university night class. Then I have trouble falling asleep afterwards!"

When we asked people how they dealt with emotionally distressed moods, they suggested a wide range of simple but effective ideas that are often thought of as clichés. Underlying these suggestions is the need to try to shift your perspective from "stuck" or "trapped" to one that helps you see choices and options ahead. Initiating small changes that make life easier is a good place to start. One woman described how getting a new telephone made a real difference. "My daughter was calling me during business hours several times a day and it was really getting me down. Finally I bought a telephone with call display. That allowed me to know when she was calling, so I could choose whether to answer her at that time or wait and call her back later. Suddenly, I felt calm again. I could ignore the interruptions and then have one good conversation with her at the end of my working day."

Here is a toolbox of ideas (and yes, clichés) that boomers said had worked for them in alleviating and reversing negative moods:

• Engage in positive activities. Get more sleep, make love, cook, do something different. Use meditation, prayer, yoga, and deep breathing to relieve stress and find inner peace. Get involved in music, art, and other creative endeavors; take time off to read. Take more vacations. Turn off the television set – "vegging there just makes things worse." Get outdoors; take a walk; get involved in aerobic exercise.
• Enjoy time with others (human and furry). Take time to enjoy the simple things in life. Spend time with your kids or grandkids. Phone

a friend. "Walk and talk" with someone who cares about you. Walk the dog; play with your kitten.
- Use humor to diffuse the pressure.
- Adopt a positive attitude. Try to "take life one day at a time," and "be grateful for what you have!" Ask yourself, "Will this really matter fifty years from now?" Recognize that things are cyclical, and they will change.
- Adjust your work schedule. Cut down on your work hours; say no. Don't bring a briefcase full of work home every night. Retire!
- Don't be afraid to seek help.

While the above list is useful for dealing with the occasional depressed mood, these strategies are not enough for dealing with more serious problems. Today, treatment for people with serious clinical depression and anxiety usually involves prescribed medication (especially the family of drugs called SSRIs – selective serotonin reuptake inhibitors – such as Prozac, Celexa, and Paxil), combined with counseling. In our survey, almost one-third had been to or were currently undergoing psychotherapy. Overall, their experiences in counseling were very positive, not only for dealing with specific problems but for taking time to reflect out loud and develop a different perspective on their lives. In a society in which "multi-tasking" is the expected norm, boomers are so busy doing that they seldom take time to just *be* and talk about their inner feelings.

Many people saw psychotherapy as a unique opportunity to claim time for their inner selves and to understand themselves better. "Psychotherapy is only partly about changing things around us," said one man. "It is also for insight, acceptance, and inner transformation." Another person said, "Counseling has helped me to look objectively at myself and freed me to really live my life."

One person said, "Counseling has helped me change my self-perception, find new skills and emotional resources, and resolve issues through letting go of previous illusions." Some talked about unresolved issues that went back to their childhoods. "I had many ghosts from my past, and I was able to release them in order to deal with my problem," said one woman. "I now understand my behavior and mentality better, and I am able to set goals for the future."

In the Healthy Boomer Midlife Survey, the top four strategies recommended for dealing with emotional stress were:

- counseling and medication;
- physical activity;
- complementary and alternative therapies such as St. John's Wort, massage, and shiatsu; and
- talking things out with family members and friends.

One man told us how a psychiatrist he knew believed that some people who use exercise to treat a depressed mood do as well as people on antidepressants. "My father had mental health problems. I like the idea of not using drugs, so I started to train for a triathlon. I have been doing it ever since, and I feel great!"

Boomers who use physical activity to help deal with emotional distress are on to something good. According to the U.S. Surgeon General's 1996 Report on Physical Activity and Health, inactive people are twice as likely to suffer symptoms of depression as more active people. Numerous studies have shown that aerobic exercise, such as running or brisk walking and sports can help lift your mood and combat depression. While exercise cannot replace medication or psychotherapy if you are severely depressed, it can help you deal with the occasional depressed mood and can be good preventive medicine. Physical activity, especially walking outdoors, can also be a beneficial complement to other treatments for people with major depression or anxiety episodes.

### Are You Getting Enough . . . Zzzz?

Fatigue, a depressed mood, anxiety, and sleep deprivation are often linked. In fact, it is difficult to know which is the chicken and which the egg. The question "Are you sleep deprived or are you depressed?" is particularly relevant for boomer women who are undergoing dramatic hormone fluctuations.

In our survey, one-third of the respondents said they suffer from insomnia – a percentage that matches larger Statistics Canada surveys of adults. "Insomnia makes me feel irritable, forgetful, and fatigued," said one person, "and it causes daytime sleepiness."

Even two nights of sleep deprivation can affect how well we function. "When insomnia strikes two nights in a row, it ruins my feelings of well-being," said one man, "and I become concerned that I will not cope as well at work." Another person noted that fatigue caused by a lack of sleep "makes for one crabby and guilty parent."

### SOME HIGHLIGHTS FROM THE HEALTHY BOOMER MIDLIFE SURVEY

| *In an average week, how many hours do you sleep each night?* | |
| --- | --- |
| More than 8 hours | 3% |
| About 8 hours | 35% |
| 5 to 7 hours | 58% |
| Less than 5 hours | 4% |

| *In an average week, how often do you wake up feeling well rested?* | |
| --- | --- |
| 7 of 7 nights | 9% |
| 5 or 6 of 7 nights | 40% |
| 3 or 4 of 7 nights | 28% |
| 1 or 2 of 7 nights | 18% |
| 0 out of 7 nights | 5% |

Most sleep experts recommend getting eight hours of sleep each night. In our survey, the majority (57%) said they get five to seven hours of sleep a night; 38 per cent got eight hours or more. But the quality of sleep may be more important than the actual quantity. Only 9 per cent claimed they wake feeling rested each morning. Almost one-third reported they wake up feeling rested only three to four days each week.

Some people identified their main problem as an inability to stay asleep, not getting to sleep in the first place. Physical changes in midlife may be part of the reason. In many cases, midlife women are awakened by hot flashes, and sometimes severe night sweats. Their thrashing and discomfort may waken their partners. Conversely, midlife men talked about the need to get up to urinate in the night – sometimes several times – and how this often woke their partners. Women with hot flashes found that using hormone replacement therapy (HRT) and having a thin, soft sheet as the first layer on the bed helped. Men mentioned the importance of drinking no beverages in the evening, especially alcohol.

A recent study among midlife adults who had sleep-maintenance problems (in *Informed 2001*, a newsletter from the Institute for Clinical Evaluative Sciences) showed that the following strategies also help:

- Establish a standard wake-up time seven days a week.
- Get out of bed if you do not quickly fall back to sleep. Go to another room to read, or listen to music and/or have a cup of warm milk with honey. After you start to feel drowsy, go back to bed.
- Avoid non-sleeping activities in the bedroom, including reading and watching television.
- Eliminate daytime napping.

Bed partners in midlife are well aware of each other's problems with sleep and mood, which may be associated with menopause in women and andropause in men. Some 30 per cent of both sexes cited sleep disturbances as a sign of male menopause, or andropause, and more than 40 per cent cited sleep disturbances as a problem in female menopause. "It is difficult to stay emotionally stable when you have poor sleep patterns," said one woman. "I need to recognize my mood is a symptom of my fatigue and deal with it appropriately."

### From the Research
*Thinking Positively about Mental Fitness*
Research at Simon Fraser University has shown that positive beliefs about the potential for growth in later life helped people from ages fifty to ninety-one improve their mental fitness and, in some cases, their memories. Participants in one-day workshops learned to turn negative beliefs about their declining mental abilities into positive ones. They learned how to think and act creatively, to appreciate differing views, and to listen to each other with renewed respect. All reported dramatic increases in their level of mental fitness.
Source: Crusack, S. A., and W. J. A. Thompson. *International Journal of Lifelong Education* (1998), as reported in *JAMA*, Vol. 285, No. 11 (March 21, 2001).

*Depression and Smoking*
A recent analysis by Statistics Canada has shown that people who smoke have increased odds of having major depressive episodes, compared with non-smokers. The odds were almost double for men and, for women, one-and-a-half times greater. It is not yet clear why this is so. The authors of the study suggest that depression-prone people may use tobacco to self-medicate, or that tobacco use and depression may share some common genetic basis.
Source: Statistics Canada. "Psychological Health – Depression," *Health Reports*, Vol. 11, No. 3 (Winter, 1999).

## On the Lighter Side
We think that all of you who worry and laugh about your memory lapses – as we do – will enjoy this story that a friend sent by e-mail.

*Hallelujah and Amen*
A middle-aged man bought a donkey from a preacher. The preacher told the man that this donkey had been trained in a unique way. The only way to make the donkey go was to say "Hallelujah!" The way to make him stop was to say "Amen."

The man was pleased with his purchase and immediately got on the animal to try out the preacher's instructions. "Hallelujah!" shouted the man. The donkey began to trot. "Amen!" shouted the man. The donkey stopped immediately. "This is great!" said the man.

With a "Hallelujah," he rode off on his new purchase. The man traveled for a long time through some mountains. Soon he realized he was heading towards a cliff. Then he realized he could not remember the word to make the donkey stop. "Stop," he said. "Halt!" he cried. The donkey just kept on going.

"Oh no!" "Bible!" "Church!" "Please stop!" shouted the man. The donkey just began to trot faster. He was getting closer and closer to the edge of the cliff. Finally in desperation, the man said a prayer, "Please, dear Lord, please make this donkey stop before I go over the edge of this mountain. In *JESUS*' name, Amen."

The donkey came to an abrupt stop just one step from the edge of the cliff.

"Hallelujah!" shouted the man.

## Questions to Reflect On

Emotional health is a critical component of our overall well-being. It is closely linked with wellness and illness in the body.

1.  When you think of your overall well-being, do you factor in your emotional health? Do you put as much effort into enhancing your emotional well-being as you do your physical health?
2.  When you have a physical concern, such as a headache, backache, or indigestion, do you take time to consider whether it is linked to an emotional upset?
3.  Do you think you deny emotional distress in your life? For example, do you self-medicate with alcohol, drugs, or excess work?
4.  What is one area of your emotional health that needs shoring up?
5.  What is one simple, specific thing you can do today to take care of your inner self (e.g., call a friend, go to a movie, take a walk)?
6.  Do you honestly wake up feeling rested? If not, what is one small change you could make to improve your sleep (e.g., turn off all the lights in the house ten minutes earlier)?

# CHAPTER TWO

# Shifting Focus:
# Making Changes That Last

Not everything that is faced can be changed, but nothing can be changed until it is faced.

— James A. Baldwin, 1924–1987

We don't like change. Sure, we would like to weigh 130 pounds instead of 160. We want to be able to hike without feeling our lungs will burst. But what we don't want to do is get up in the morning when we're tired and worried about money or last night's argument, cheerfully don running shoes, and go out there to embrace the new day. Like all human beings, we want to be magically changed in the desired ways with minimal effort on our part. This applies to all kinds of changes, both physical and emotional. In psychotherapy, it is not unusual to hear people say "This is not working for me" after only a few sessions – as if they were taking the car in for a tune-up and wanted the quickest service at the cheapest price.

This chapter addresses the process of change, primarily by explaining a stages-of-change model developed in 1994 by psychologist James Prochaska and his colleagues John Norcross and Carlo DiClemente. While it is theoretical in nature, we have tried to present it in a practical way. It will help you to understand change and to succeed in your efforts to make personal changes in all areas of your life. We hope that you will keep the model in mind as you work your way through the other chapters in this book.

## Blame It on Our Old Reptilian Brains

It's not so much that we're lazy. It's just that our physiological selves crave homeostasis. In the oldest, reptilian part of our brains, no change is good change. No change means safety and security, and that is important above all else. Yes, very sophisticated areas of our brains are capable of amazingly complex creative thought patterns. But when push comes to shove, the old reptile in us just wants to eat something, belch, and go back to sleep. Hence, we have the rows and rows of self-help books in the local bookstore, the motivational tapes and seminars, the popularity of Oprah and Rosie and Dr. Phil. We are always trying to prod, cajole, threaten, flatter, and beg the old reptile to take up the tango or weight training or yoga. He or she just yawns and grunts and looks the other way.

Because change is difficult, there is no one approach that works all the time or for all people. Too often we get discouraged and stop trying, not because we really can't change but because we are unrealistic – both in our expectations of ourselves and in our notions of how change happens. This is why we need a range of options to get us started and keep us going.

That said, many people have told us that they have been able to make significant life changes that have radically altered how they feel about themselves. A fifty-three-year-old lawyer who was inspired by both a new partner and a health scare said, "I finally did it. I lost thirty pounds. It took me more than three years to do it, but I feel great." Obviously, change does not happen overnight or without a lot of concentrated effort.

When James Prochaska and his colleagues studied the process of personal change, they divided it into a series of steps. Understanding that change is a process comprising a number of steps or stages, knowing what these are, and determining where you are at any point in the process can be a strong incentive to going on when you hit that wall that says you can't do it. Here is our version of the model developed by Prochaska.

**The Stages of Change**
There are five stages:

1. Precontemplation
2. Contemplation
3. Preparation
4. Action
5. Maintenance

As you read through these stages, remember that the process is not a linear one. You will spend longer in some stages than others, and you will move through some of the stages a few or many times. This does not mean that you are failing. This is the way the process works.

The biggest mistake most people make is to leap immediately to the action stage. We will therefore spend more time talking about the first three stages, in which our reptilian brains need the most persuading.

THE STAGES OF CHANGE MODEL

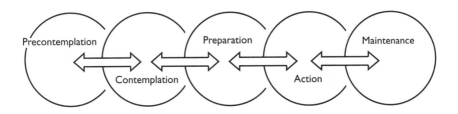

*Resisting Change – Precontemplation*

If contemplation is the state of beginning to think about and ponder something, then precontemplation is that hazy, ill-defined period that comes before. It goes like this: "Someday, sometime, I should take a look at maybe thinking about cutting down on my drinking a little. But I have to go to a cocktail party tonight and I don't drink too much anyway." At this stage, people don't see the problem, let alone a solution.

In the precontemplation stage, we strongly resist even acknowledging there is something we should change. The old reptilian brain is in full command. Our minds are full of all the reasons why it is too difficult to do something or why we really don't need to do it anyway. Again and again we hear in the clinic: "I've tried everything and nothing works"; "Maybe I'm just one of those people who can't quit"; "I just don't have the willpower"; "I don't have time to deal with this now."

Here are some other ways you can tell that you are in this stage:

- Family, friends, and colleagues keep saying they see a problem and you don't.
- You think they're the ones who should change, not you.
- You don't really have that much information about whatever the issue is, and you kind of like it that way.

- You feel demoralized and believe the situation is hopeless at times.
- You don't want to take responsibility for this problem.

Resistance, which is defined as "refusal to comply," is at its strongest in this stage. Often, we misunderstand resistance, seeing it as a rock-hard impediment to moving ahead – one that means we should give up. Here is how a forty-year-old woman put it:

"I am feeling really frustrated that I constantly keep dealing with the same stuff over and over again. I just wish that people were like cars. The brakes are broken? No problem, get them fixed. No such luck. Always working, working, working at making changes and trying to understand my way of thinking and why it is not easier. I just do not seem to get past the bad habits. I know I have to change for the sake of my health, but that seems to make me even more frustrated and sometimes I don't care as much. . . . I just do not have the motivation! I feel it's never going to change, so what is the point of trying?"

Fortunately, this resistance can help us be discerning and thoughtful about what we are doing. To change means to give up something familiar to us. Starting to walk every evening means giving up the couch-potato time and the rituals associated with it that we have come to equate with relaxation. Starting to eat in a more healthful way may mean giving up some of those special desserts that remind us of the comforts of childhood.

Most of us experience a sense of loss when we give up an old behavior or addiction – no matter how rationally we know we need to change it – because we are then giving up a certain way that we know ourselves. We don't like to do that, so we resist. Yet it is part of the paradox of human change that, when we can say to ourselves, "I'm resisting doing something better for myself," we are in fact taking an important step in consciously acknowledging where we are. We are already in the process of changing. Being conscious of where we are helps us move on to some other place. No matter how precise the directions are for telling you how to get from Sudbury to North Bay, if you don't know where you are now in relation to Sudbury you don't have a chance.

Some people stay in the precontemplation stage for years or decades or even a lifetime. Often, a significant birthday, such as turning forty or fifty, can trigger inward movement toward the next stage. Other catalysts for change include major events such as remarriage, the marriage of your child, the arrival of grandchildren, impending retirement, and especially a brush with serious illness or the death of a close friend. Often something quite dramatic rather than the accumulation of little nudges propels us in the direction of action.

What can help you move to the next stage? Most of all, it seems to be a combination of these three factors:

- facing and dealing with your resistance to change;
- becoming more knowledgeable about your self-defeating behavior;
- obtaining support from others who do not nag but clearly acknowledge the problem.

Learn a little bit more about your problem and how other people deal with it, and then find somebody who will support you in the change process. If you are unable to deal with resistance yourself, this can be a good time to see a psychotherapist who understands how resistance and denial operate, and can help you recognize what is holding you back. You can also seek support from your family physician, a fitness coach, an AA buddy, a friend, or family member. Keep in mind, however, that family members may have their own difficult feelings about your behavior, especially if it has had a negative impact on them. Sometimes a neutral person is best.

### The Procrastinator's Paradise – Contemplation

The difference between precontemplation and contemplation is subtle but significant. Before, you couldn't see the problem; now you can. However, you aren't quite ready to do more than think about it. This stage is a procrastinator's paradise. You have found out where you are in relation to Sudbury and you have the directions to get there, but you aren't willing to leave for North Bay just yet. So, the resistance continues. People can remain stuck here for a very long time. You acknowledge that you have a problem and begin to think seriously about solving it. You may have a general plan to do something within the next six months or so, but you are still far from making a serious commitment to action.

One of the risks here is that of becoming a chronic contemplator – that is, getting very interested in your problem in an abstract way, as if it is a problem in theory rather than in your life. You substitute thinking about the problem for action. You postpone action to some undetermined future time. For example, you say to yourself, "I can't change my diet today, I'll start on Monday. No, it would be better to start the first of the month. No, that's Jerry's birthday, and there'll be cake in the office, so maybe I'll start when we go on vacation."

As you move through this stage, the desire to change slowly grows, but it seems to exist alongside the resistance. You may feel a great deal of ambivalence and frustrated inner dialogue. "I want to stop feeling so stuck, but . . ." and then out come all the reasons not to do anything. This is because taking action to change a comforting, familiar behavior, however self-destructive it may appear to the outsider, is quite terrifying for the old reptilian brain. The familiar self is still safer and more desirable than a better, healthier self.

Here are a few of the traps that interfere with moving on:

- The search for absolute certainty (believing you must "perfectly" understand your problem first);
- Magical thinking (believing that there is a magic or perfect time to take action);
- Wishful thinking (for example, "If only I could eat whatever I wanted and not gain weight");
- Premature action (taking action without being ready). This can cause a serious setback that will delay moving forward even longer.

When the prospects for change stall in the contemplation stage, it is easy for us to become disheartened and resigned to the status quo. Here is what the research says can help us move on:

*Get in touch with your feelings.* It helps a lot to get emotionally charged about the need to change. This could take the form of excitement about the prospect of a yearned-for hiking trip if you lose ten pounds. It could be the fear of a heart attack, because your brother just had one, or anger that you're not able to do things you used to do. The feeling must be strong enough to motivate you but not so strong that it becomes incapacitating. An intellectual interest in your problem without an emotional charge keeps you in the contemplation stage.

*Define your goals.* Be specific rather than vague about what you want to do. Set an agenda for yourself, rather than being dictated to by others. For example, "I want to walk three times a week," rather than "I want to be more fit and healthy."

*Monitor your behavior on an ongoing basis.* Be precise. For example, decide how many calories or how many drinks you will consume and count how many you actually have each day. Identify what immediately precedes a problem behavior and what follows it, both in terms of what you do and how you feel. Is there inner self-talk that justifies your problem, such as, "After all I've done today, I deserve this"? What is the payoff for the self-defeating actions? There is always a payoff, even if it is not immediately apparent. Is there some sense of freedom or adolescent rebellion? "I can do what I want! No one is going to tell me what to do!" It is difficult but crucial to observe and monitor your behaviors in as unbiased way, as free of judgments as possible. Think of yourself as a researcher, collecting data about this very interesting subject – you. Passing judgment on what you are doing or how you are feeling guarantees prolonged stuckness!

Many people who get stuck at this stage believe they know all there is to know and still can't move beyond this point. This is often not the case. What they know, they know very, very well. The problem is that of being open to different ways of looking at where and how they are stuck. Working with the three directives listed above may require a psychotherapist's help, especially if the behavior you are trying to change is particularly long-standing or especially self-destructive. Eventually, you want to accumulate a critical mass of knowledge and information, become more aware of your own thought processes, and increase your self-motivation with activated emotion, so that you can move on to the next stage.

It is also important in this stage to begin to develop a process of self-evaluation. This means honestly looking at how things really are. For example, "I really smoked sixteen cigarettes today," or "I really did lose count of the number of times I yelled at my kids today, and only said two supportive things." Self-evaluation is useful when it involves the following three behaviors:

1.  Take time to think before you engage in behavior that doesn't work for you. For example, "If my spouse is not a morning person, why do I keep picking the morning to try to have an important conversation?"
2.  Imagine yourself without the negative behavior. See yourself playing the violin you've always dreamed about or hiking a mountain path. Visualization, which is used by all high-performance athletes, is most useful when there is a great deal of sensory detail. Include the smells, sounds, feel, and tastes of a particular scene.
3.  Make a decision. Evaluate the pros and cons of changing your behavior in terms of the consequences of this change to you and to others. Whether or not you can then make a decision is key to determining whether you can then move to the preparation stage.

At this point, it is most helpful for others to acknowledge your effort ("I know you'll do your best"), rather than being judgmental ("Oh no, you're doing that again!") or responding with a sense of false confidence ("Of course you'll do it!").

*Getting Ready – Preparation*
Preparation, or "getting ready," is the third important stage in the process of change. Imagine for a moment that you are going on a holiday. The precontemplation script would run like this: "We should go to Vancouver sometime to see Aunt Mary, but I guess it won't be this year." The contemplation stage script would be: "We really should do it. We could go in June, when I have some extra holidays to use. This could be exciting. You call her and I'll call the travel agent." Preparation is booking the ticket and starting to pack your bags. Obviously, the trip will be a lot more enjoyable and you'll be better able to handle unexpected challenges if you have made careful and thoughtful preparation, rather than just jumped on the plane. This stage takes you from the decisions you made in the contemplation stage into the specific steps you need to make in order to take action successfully.

This stage is also about continuing to work at resolving the ambivalence you have about changing. It is about increasing your commitment to the possibility of change. These elements are key to success at this stage:

- Continue the self-evaluation you have started. A hopeful vision of what life will be like with this changed behavior can be motivating.
- Work at increasing your confidence in your ability to change – "I can do it!"
- Increase your focus on future possibilities and less on problems of the past.
- Take small steps. Setting a date for action prevents both premature action and prolonged procrastination.
- Create your own unique action plan.
- Go public. This is always more powerful than a private pledge to yourself.
- Prepare as if for a major operation. This is a kind of psychic surgery, as you move away from allowing the reptilian brain to take charge!
- Knowing that change is not easy, have available your toolbox of techniques for coping with the barriers to change.

In a way, the preparation stage is like a rehearsal. It can feel tedious when we just want a magical solution and not all this concentrated work. It's a risky point in the process, because we may want to "just go for it." We risk falling flat on our noses, feeling sorry for ourselves, and retreating. Olympic athletes prepare by practicing countless hours week after week, year after year, to reach their goals. Why should it be different for the rest of us?

**Marianne** described her process of change: "I always wanted to row, even when I was young. My family physician kept encouraging me to get in shape and lose weight. Finally, I decided I would try rowing. I was too embarrassed to do it alone, so I asked a friend to come with me. Rowing completely changed my life! My friend quit after about two weeks, but I stuck it out. I was there with all these young people, and I felt old and fat. But they were nice to me and I kept going. I now train once a week. I work out to get stronger. I see a nutritionist, not to lose weight but to have energy to row. I deal with stress better, and even though I lost my mother this year I coped much better with the grief. I lost weight once before, in the eighties, but it is very different now. I love rowing!"

Marianne prepared herself in a way that led to healthy action. She was motivated to become more active through her relationship with her family physician. She chose an activity that she had loved when she was younger, and she enlisted the support of a friend to get started.

*Moving On – Action*

"I finally got out walking three evenings in a row and I feel like I've got it made. I'm a walker now! I did it! But then there was Jeff's baseball practice on Wednesday night and Sue's birthday dinner on Thursday and that project deadline. Before I knew it, a month had gone by since my last evening walk." Sound familiar? The action stage is the one we all want to reach. But if we have unrealistic expectations and are not properly prepared for it, it is often the one that causes the most trouble.

It would be unreasonable to expect to play the *Moonlight Sonata* after a month of piano lessons, but somehow we do expect to change lifelong patterns with little or no practice or preparation. Failing as a result of these unrealistic expectations demoralizes us. The "more of the same" approach also defeats us. This is when we hold onto the same old techniques that brought us some success in the past. In the action phase, as in all the other stages, using a variety of techniques at different times is most likely to lead to success.

Beware the temptation to equate action with the whole process of change. This negates both the critical work involved in preparing for successful action and the equally important and often more challenging efforts needed to maintain these changes. Remind yourself that action is neither the first nor the last step in the cycle. Action without preparation rarely lasts more than a day or two.

Here are some useful techniques once you have started to take action:

- Substitute healthy responses for problem behaviors wherever you can (e.g., meet a friend for a walk instead of a coffee).
- Practice substitution in your head as well. Whenever you become aware of troubling thoughts, acknowledge that they are not helpful and replace them with more positive ones.

- Use healthy diversions. Refocus your energy on an activity that precludes problem behavior (e.g., go swimming with friends – it is hard to smoke when you are doing laps!)
- Reinforce your actions with relaxation activities that help you breathe deeply and become calmer. Change can lead to a lot of anxiety.
- Avoid places you associate with the problem behavior (e.g., go to a healthy ethnic take-out restaurant rather than a hamburger fast-food place).
- Give yourself reminders of the behavior you want to reinforce (e.g., put signs on your bathroom mirror reminding you to say positive things to your children each day).
- Reward yourself in very specific ways (e.g., get a pedicure once you reach your goal of walking three times a week for four weeks).

Once again, it is important to remember that these techniques are not useful in starting a process of change, but they can be very helpful in reinforcing the action phase, when you can build on well-practiced, well-rewarded earlier steps.

We are all addicted in our own ways to our unhealthy behaviors. They are familiar and comfortable to us. Changes can bring with them unexpected anxiety, fear, and uncertainty. "Why should I be feeling anxious when I'm doing something good for myself?" Remember that old reptilian brain for which no change is good. The disequilibrium that comes with change can feel like a threat, and therefore is countered with all the resistance that can be mustered. This is why it is important to use all the ways and means at your disposal to ease your passage towards new and healthier habits.

In this phase, support people are most helpful when they are dependable and acknowledge both the effort required of you and the gains you are making. This is a great time to have a buddy. When we support someone who also supports us, we find the positive reinforcement increases exponentially!

### Staying There – Maintenance

Maintenance is long, active, and ongoing. This is the stage of working to consolidate the gains you have made and to minimize and prevent lapses and relapses. The greatest challenges to maintaining changes are:

- overconfidence (e.g., getting lulled into thinking it was easy);
- daily temptations (e.g., to have that one drink or one dessert);
- self-blame and criticizing oneself for any slight lapse.

In the maintenance phase, it is important to continue to use the Stages of Change model to see where you are in the process, and to experiment with different ways of supporting the change. Continue to use all the methods that helped you reach the action stage. Here are some of the techniques people find most helpful at this stage:

- Keep a healthy distance from people, places, and things that could seriously compromise your change, especially during the early months. During maintenance, as in the action stage, commitment is not enough. It must be coupled with supportive environments.
- Work to create alternative behaviors, such as a healthier lifestyle. This is one of the most important challenges of maintenance.
- Check regularly how you are thinking about the change you have made. Be honest with yourself. Remind yourself why you needed to make the change and what obstacles you have faced.
- Be patient with yourself and persistent.
- Helping someone else can reinforce your own changes.

Fifty-five year-old **Helen**, who is now maintaining a regular physical-activity regimen, said to her family physician, "I cannot believe how stubborn and resistant I was. I remember everything you used to tell me, that there was more to life than my work. I could not see how money fears and work pressures controlled my life. I did not understand then, but I do now. I finally got it. I know what is important now."

### Lapses – One Slip Does Not Make a Fall

Lapses are inevitable for just about everybody. But many people give up as soon as they lapse, because they hold mistaken beliefs. They see the lapse as a total failure or think that it means the process was totally wrong. In fact, what led to the lapse and how they responded to it may provide valuable information about what they may need to do differently to maintain the change. To view lapses as failures or as "falling off the wagon" or as "starting all over again" can mean a return to the contemplation stage in which they just think about doing something and don't act.

Ask yourself these questions at this point:

- Is my drive to change waning?
- How can I get back on track – from Contemplation back to Preparation and Action?
- How can I strengthen my desire to make this change?

Finally, Prochaska and DiClemente write about a termination stage, wherein you exit the cycle of change. At this point, you no longer experience temptation in any situation and your new behavior is totally solid. The problem with this idea is that it precludes changes in your life that make us all susceptible to falling back into the old negative patterns. It seems to work better for most people to think of themselves as continuing in a maintenance mode, which may continue to need more or less shoring up, depending on their current stress levels and circumstances.

### The Bottom Line

When we asked respondents to the Healthy Boomer Midlife Survey what one change they would most like to make in the next year, about half said they would like to make changes to their physical health. The other half wanted to make changes in their emotional and spiritual health (see Introduction and Chapters 1 and 13) and in their relationships (see Chapters 8, 9, and 10). Others noted some very specific changes they would like to make in the year to come.

- "I want to get rid of my blood-pressure pills and get better erections."
- "I want to find time to go on daily walks, which I like to do."
- "I want to get rid of my bloated stomach and wrinkles!"
- "I want to be more positive with my kids."
- "I want to spend more time with my mother before she dies."

What was most striking was that these people did not strive for bigger houses or fancy cars. Their wishes were modest and, for the most part, they were looking for ways to better balance their physical, mental, and spiritual well-being. With an increased awareness of their mortality, the boomers are looking to get off the treadmill of daily responsibilities and to make lasting personal changes that nourish the self and give something back to others. When we make this shift and recognize what makes us restless and unhappy and open our eyes to the possibility of a change, the process can begin.

We hope that a better understanding of the process of personal change will be helpful as you read the rest of this book. As you reflect on areas of your life that you would like to change, keep the following points in mind:

- Choose something specific and manageable that you really want to change, not your whole life all at once.
- Remember that this is a process in which one moves back and forth between stages for quite a while.
- The time a change takes is totally individual, and depends on factors such as how long the negative pattern has been in place, the strength of your drive to change, the amount of support you have from other people and in your particular environment, and your general level of stress.
- Get and give support.
- Lapses are not failures. They are a critical part of the learning curve.
- Get professional help when you need it.

### From the Research
Recently, a group of prominent behavioral scientists endorsed eight conditions, all of which must be true if a person is to effectively change a behavior:

1. The person has formed a strong positive intention to perform the behavior.
2. There are no environmental barriers that make it impossible for the behavior to occur.
3. The person has the skills necessary to perform the behavior.

4. The person believes the advantages of performing the behavior out-weigh the disadvantages.
5. The person perceives more social pressure to perform than to not perform the behavior.
6. The person perceives that the behavior is consistent with his or her self-image and does not violate personal standards.
7. The person's emotional reaction to performing the behavior is more positive than negative.
8. The person has the perceived self-efficacy (belief in her or his ability to succeed) to execute the behavior.

Source: National Institutes of Health, National Cancer Institute (U.S.). *Theory at a Glance: A Guide for Health Promotion Practice, 2001.*
http://rex.nci.nih.gov/NCI_Pub_Interface/Theory_at_glance/HOME.html

**On the Lighter Side**
Q. How many psychologists does it take to change a light bulb?
A. Only one, but the light bulb has to really want to change.

*Baby Boomers Then and Now*
1970: long hair
2000: longing for hair

1970: acid rock
2000: acid reflux

1970: moving to California because it's cool
2000: moving to California because it's warm

1970: growing pot
2000: growing pot belly

1970: watching John Glenn's historic space flight with your parents
2000: watching John Glenn's historic space flight with your children

1970: hoping for a BMW
2000: hoping for a BM

1970: getting your head stoned
2000: getting your headstone

1970: getting out to a new hip joint
2000: getting a new hip joint

## Questions to Reflect On

1. What is one change you would like to make, using the process of change model described in this chapter?
2. What is one specific step you can take now to move from thinking about it (Contemplation) to getting ready (Preparation)?
3. Who can you realistically ask to support you in this change?

# CHAPTER THREE

# *The Balancing Act*

Every morning you are handed twenty-four golden hours. They are one of the few things in this world that you get free of charge. If you had all the money in the world, you couldn't buy an extra hour. What will you do with this priceless treasure? Remember, you must use it, as it is given only once. Once wasted you cannot get it back.

— Author Unknown

"I know what I should be doing, but I don't have the time!"

"I just don't have the energy to cook a healthy meal when I get home from work."

"I feel like I have lost the sense of joy in my life."

These are the familiar refrains we heard over and over from men and women in midlife. We know we need to go swimming with the kids, visit friends, meditate, take time with our partners, do our back exercises, finish work projects, visit our mothers, or just sit quietly to watch the clouds go by. But overburdened with midlife responsibilities and a perception that we need to do it all, we are unable to find time to take care of ourselves. Rushing anxiously from task to task, we often fail to see that we do, in fact, have those precious twenty-four hours each day, and that we also have a choice in how we spend them.

Boomers repeatedly claim that a lack of time and energy are the key barriers to their establishing a better balance in their lives, and to reclaiming the sense of joy that they miss. This chapter explores these issues and offers some suggestions from our peers and other experts on how to create time, energy, and joy in midlife. It also includes an exercise you can use to decide how you would like to adjust the current balance in your life among hours spent on body, mind, spirit, work, and play.

## The Boomers' Time-and-Energy Crunch

"It makes me crazy that this is the only time that I will be middle-aged," said one woman, "and I just don't have the energy to take advantage of all the joys and opportunities without feeling completely overwhelmed."

When we come home from work exhausted, only to face a second job of household duties and family responsibilities, often we are too spent to know what to do first. Boomers tell us repeatedly what a struggle it is to live with so much pressure. They feel overwhelmed and guilty because they can't do it all. After all, we should help our aging parents more, spend more time with our children, and share more meaningful time with our partners. And then there is the lunch or dinner with a close friend that has been postponed for the third time. When confronted with all of these responsibilities at the same time, we lose sight of the fact that each of these connections can be satisfying and joyful in its own right. The mix seems to sour, and we end up feeling battered and depleted instead.

We are a society that is increasingly addicted to being in a stressed state. This means that it feels normal to be constantly stressed and abnormal when we are not moving at a frantic pace. We sign up for spiritual retreats and yoga and Pilates classes in an effort to slow down and renew ourselves. The danger is that we will approach these activities with the same frenetic energy, and make them part of an endless and ultimately fruitless search – just one more thing to let us down.

When "there is no time for me," we often end up denying how we feel. The high-stress state we live in begins to manifest itself in physical symptoms, such as chronic tiredness, heartburn, indigestion, and all-over aching. Chronic fatigue syndrome, fibromyalgia, and other conditions that are rooted in the body and the psyche become more common in this overburdened world. As one forty-five-year-old woman said, "I cannot understand this! I feel tired all the time. I am dizzy. I have indigestion and feel weak. I should not be feeling like this; there must be something wrong!"

Most of the time, we are responsible, loving people. In the face of constant stress, however, we often don't respond in kind and loving ways to the people who matter the most. "I do not even remember the last time my wife and I made love," said one man. "We work hard and come home tired late at night. By the time we cook dinner, eat, and have a glass of wine, usually

I just pass out. When I do take time off, I go to visit my sick mother in England. Last weekend we finally took a thirty-six-hour weekend off from work. We drove to Niagara-on-the-Lake, but we ended up sleeping in, because we were totally exhausted."

"We are a nation in love with speed," writes Jeremy Rifkin in his book *Time Wars* (1987). He says, "We have become more organized but less spontaneous, less joyful. Time itself, of course, has not speeded up; it's our perception of time that has moved us into high gear."

On the surface of things, the explanation for how we got here is fairly simple. We are working longer hours than ever before. We have cultivated a society that promotes constant hurrying as a way to produce more and get more done, although we can't necessarily say why this is so. New technologies such as the Internet, e-mail, and cell phones have upped the pace of information transfer and made us available all hours of the day and night. We are no longer in control of our own time. As we race the clock to keep up, we lose the ability to think about basic values and what we really want in life. Our lack of insight into the stress that time pressures create in our personal lives and in our relationships only makes us feel worse.

Many boomers try to manage time as if it were a commodity we can manipulate and abuse, while hoping there will be some huge amount of it later on, in some place called "retirement." We assume that we will know how to enjoy that time, even though we haven't practiced having time on our hands for decades. No wonder we see newly retired people moving at the same frenetic pace – but this time at playful activities. Like the alcoholic who denies how many drinks she has had, we deny the reality that time will win out in the end, that time will go on long after we have stopped. Perhaps the poets say it best. It is Shakespeare's Richard II who speaks the famous line "I wasted time, and now doth time waste me."

### Dealing with Time Sickness

Why is it that many boomers, who are innovative and organized in their work, suddenly become paralyzed when it comes to applying the same energy and knowledge to organizing time for themselves? We wish there were a simple solution to this dilemma, but there isn't. If this frantic level of being in the world is what the reptilian brain has been trained to accept

as "normal," change will not be easy. But change it we can – slowly, awk-
wardly, and one small step at a time.

Here are some strategies for preventing and healing time sickness.

*Put Time in Perspective*
There is no doubt that many boomers face enormous external pressures
related to work and family. However, in our clinic and seminars, we often
tell people that, as long as we see ourselves as victims of time, we won't be
able to change in the ways we want to. Each of us has the same twenty-four
hours as everyone else. Imagine saying to yourself, "I am *choosing* to spend
this day trying to do more than I can, and then feeling badly afterwards."
While this may sound foolish, the point is that it is better to acknowledge
what we are doing to ourselves than to deny it. Once we are conscious of
this, we can begin to feel in charge of how we spend our time. Only then do
we have a chance to make real and lasting changes. Perspective is everything – in art and in life!

Russ Kisby, former president of ParticipACTION, describes a unique
way to put time in perspective that formed the basis of a popular motivational campaign to get Canadians more active. "There are 1,440 minutes in

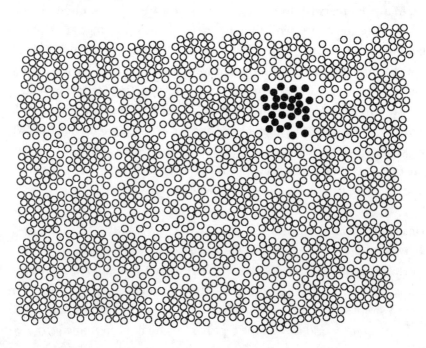

a day," says Russ. "If you were to make 1,440 dots on a page and highlight just 30 of them, it would not seem like very much. But that is all it takes. For example, spending 30 minutes each day walking with a dog could mean enormous benefits to your physical, emotional, and social health."

*Stop Trying to Do It All*

We seem to have become a generation of adrenaline junkies. How many times do we read and hear about all the things we should be buying to make life easier, or doing, to improve our physical health and our lives in general? Eat well, floss, get a mammogram, lift weights three times a week, go on retreat, get enough sleep, take time for yourself . . . the list goes on and on. Some people refuse to acknowledge that what they do and don't do has a profound effect on their energy levels and health problems. Others, like many conscientious boomers, go in the opposite direction, trying to change everything all at once. This is the New Year's Day Syndrome, when people decide to lose twenty pounds, get in shape, change their eating habits, and quit drinking all at the same time. There is no question that these are worthwhile goals, but people who set themselves up in this way are doomed to failure. They have missed the essential preparation stage described in the Stages of Change model in Chapter 2. It is simply unrealistic to change everything at once and expect to sustain all that change.

The baby-boom generation has been inundated with previously unheard-of possibilities and opportunities that sometimes leave us feeling like kids let loose in a candy store. Most of our parents lived through the Depression and the Second World War. They never dreamed of having or doing what many middle-class boomers now take for granted. We flip from television station to station, choosing from more than a hundred different channels, even though we can't possibly watch and take in more than one or two channels at a time. It is as if we are denying the natural constraints of time and energy.

Do we really not have enough time and energy, or are we stubbornly refusing to acknowledge these limits? How is it that busy days at the office rush by so quickly when we are trying to do it all, whereas holidays at the beach, when we're not, seem so long, full, and satisfying?

*Pace Yourself: Prevent Psychological Repetitive Strain Injury*

Pacing may be one of the remedies for life in the stress lane. When you respond to external stresses like deadlines and work overload by pressing your personal accelerator to the floor, two things happen. You squander your energy resources and your body wears out faster. As an antidote to this, one of our respondents suggested that we all "practice plodding."

Slowing down has natural consequences – the heart rate slows, the mind calms, and one becomes more present in the moment. Refusing to slow down leads to "psychological repetitive strain injury." We do the same thing over and over and lose the ability to think creatively and act effectively.

Some concrete suggestions to bring more order to chaotic living are

- try to eat, go to bed, and exercise at regular times;
- set your watch five minutes fast to avoid running late;
- practice yoga, relax by stretching, or taking a hot bath, slow your breathing with meditation;
- start a Slow Is Beautiful campaign where you work and live.

Pacing is not about standing around and doing nothing. It's about knowing when to turn up the heat and when to let things simmer down. It's about having more gears than just overdrive. Benjamin Hoff, who wrote the *Tao of Pooh* (1982), suggests that we can all learn from Winnie the Pooh's uncanny ability to go with the flow. He writes: "While Eeyore frets and Piglet hesitates and Owl pontificates, Pooh just IS."

*Give Yourself a Break*

Why is it that, when serious illness strikes, we can let go of responsibilities for which we were indispensable only moments before? Why is it that we can take time off when something is life-threatening, but we are not able to give ourselves a break in order to prevent illness or burnout? The denial of our need to have regular rest, relaxation, and rejuvenation wreaks havoc on everyone in our lives, and points to the extent to which the boomer generation is dangerously out of control.

Taking back some control over how we spend our time and energy reserves means different things to different people. Several people who responded to the Healthy Boomer Midlife Survey told us about taking planned periods of time away from their regular lives.

One couple who both work as schoolteachers spent a year traveling in South America. They spoke nostalgically about peaceful times and exciting new experiences that left them renewed and happy to return to their work. Both acknowledged how hard it is now to make time in their schedules just to go out to dinner together. Another couple told us that what works for them is sitting down once a year and scheduling four holiday periods in their calendars. "These times are sacrosanct," the woman said. "Otherwise, it would never happen." Many of us have learned that some holiday time is acceptable; taking daily and weekly breaks seems to be much more challenging. Somehow, they need to be written indelibly in our daily agendas with the same commitment that we enter work appointments.

*Use the Stages of Change Model*
One of the major challenges for people who feel they have no time or energy is to learn how to reframe their experience from the passive "I have no control" to the active "I can begin to take charge." Understanding the change model described in Chapter 2 and knowing that many people have successfully used it can be part of your preparing to reclaim some control. The model provides a structured progression through stages of change that can be reassuring. It reminds us that we can learn to walk, even if we only learned to crawl before, that falling down is a part of learning, and that there is eventually some pleasure and pride in realizing that we can get up and try again.

**What Happened to Joy?**
Joy fills the heart with gladness and delight. Young children embody it the best and often evoke it in us the most. Joy can be in a sunset, a memory, a kiss, a friend's hug, a spring morning, a song from long ago; but it must first be in us – in our hearts and in our bodies – before we can find it "out there." If we are running frantically from one meeting to another, while checking our voice mail and our e-mail and wondering whose turn it is to pick up the kids and what's for dinner, there is not much space for joy.

Joy is closely connected to time and energy. Without time and energy, there is no joy. Thus, the strategies to help us take charge of how we spend our time and use our energy are also strategies for reclaiming our joy.

Lightening up is a key step on the road to more joy. One can't "hunker down and work" at joy. Instead, one has to go in the direction of lightness, laughter, and play.

Our survey respondents repeatedly identified humor and "lightening up" as essential time-and-energy expanders. In part, this is because laughing is good for our physical and mental health. It brings more oxygen to our brains, reduces our blood pressure, and stimulates pleasurable feelings. Like exercise, if laughter could be put into a pill, it would be the most prescribed medicine for a multitude of ills.

Humor is a powerful strategy for coping under pressure, as ten years of M\*A\*S\*H and another decade of reruns have so effectively shown. Comedy writer C. W. Metcalfe suggests, in his book *Lighten Up!* (1993), that in challenging situations we adopt the credo "When the going gets tough, the tough lighten up." By assuming control over our perspective on change, we can remain creative under pressure.

Putting fun back in your life sometimes means taking the chance that you may be found wanting, even a little foolish. Writer and humorist **Anne Hines** writes in *Canadian Living* magazine (November 1998) about the time she went to a climbing gym. "Not quite Everest," she says, "but when I was six metres above the floor hanging by my fingernails, the difference seemed insignificant. My twenty-year-old instructor, Skip, kept yelling up, 'Work from your stomach muscles.' I don't have stomach muscles. I traded them eleven years ago for children."

Anne Hines talked with us about humor and aging. She says, "There is optimism and hope in humor that helps us age gracefully, especially when people go through a period of extreme stress, such as a marriage breakup. Aging with humor means respecting yourself. It's okay to have fun with the changes in our appearance that we hate, but the bottom line is accepting it and recognizing our life journey."

Playfulness, like humor, is also a way to exercise and stretch our capacity for joy. This may mean spending time with four-year-olds, who are almost always eager and engaging playmates. It may mean participating in a favorite sport, reminiscing about funny family stories with an elderly auntie, or watching reruns of *I Love Lucy*. For some it means clowning, being zany, or e-mailing your favorite cartoons or jokes to a friend.

However you evoke playfulness and humor in your life, it plants you firmly in the present moment.

We asked Anne what serious boomers could do to put some playfulness back in their lives: "Sit down and make a list of some occupations you would have liked to pursue in another life. Then go out and do something outside your regular routine that mimics that job. For example, if you always dreamed of being a country-and-western singer, go to a karaoke bar with some friends and sing your heart out. If you want to be a dancer in your next life, join a group that puts on a dance show. Don't just quietly take dance lessons. To really have fun you sometimes have to scare yourself a little!"

**Finding Your Balance**

Here is a simple exercise to show you where you currently spend your energy and time, and to help you reflect on how you would like to adjust the balance in your life.

**Circle 1** shows an equal division of time and energy in five areas of life – body, mind, spirit, work, and play. This is *not* meant to be a model of how things should be.

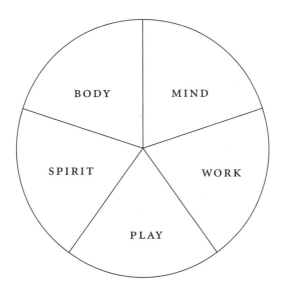

**Circle 2** is left open so that you can draw in how you currently spend your time and energy. Take a couple of deep breaths and, without thinking about it too much, draw the five segments as they best represent where you are right now.

**Circle 3** is also open for you. Draw in it how you would realistically like to change the division of your time and energy in the five areas of your life.

- Start by taking a few breaths, and do the exercise without censoring your thoughts. The first thing that comes to mind is usually what is the truest for you.
- Now, choose one of the five areas to which you want to allocate some more time and energy.
- Focus on one specific small change you can make in that area. For example, if you need to have more fun, plan an outing to the zoo with some children. Be specific. Plan a time to go, and make a commitment to carry it through.

Each of the five areas of the circle is discussed in different chapters of this book. We hope you will refer to these chapters for help in finding some specific strategies that will help you move toward change.

### From the Research
- Medical studies show that laughter boosts levels of endorphins, the body's natural painkillers, and suppresses levels of epinephrine, the stress hormone.
- In his book *Anatomy of an Illness* (1981), Norman Cousins tells how watching comedies helped him recover from an illness that he had been told would be fatal. He is generally credited with starting the scientific study of the effect of humor on physical health some twenty years ago.
- Adults laugh approximately fifteen times per day while children laugh about four hundred times per day.
- One researcher says that twenty seconds of guffawing gives the heart the same workout as three minutes' of hard rowing.

Source: Sowell, C. "Is Laughter the Best Medicine?" *QUEST*, Vol. 3, No. 4 (1996).

### On the Lighter Side
*About Midlife*
- In midlife, we learn that work is good, but it's not that important.
- Midlife means that you become more reflective. You start pondering the "big" questions. What is life? Why am I here? How much Healthy Choice ice cream can I eat before it's no longer a healthy choice?

- But midlife also brings with it an appreciation for what is important. We realize that waists expand and chins double, but our loved ones make the journey worthwhile.
- Would any of you trade the knowledge that you have now for the body you had back then? Maybe our bodies simply have to expand to hold all of the wisdom and love we've acquired . . . that's our philosophy and we're sticking to it!

### Questions to Reflect On

When we succumb to time pressures that demoralize us and drain our energy, we are in danger of losing our balance and our sense of joy in life. While we cannot always change or divert external pressures, we can take control over our time by pacing ourselves, setting priorities in our choices about change in our lives, preparing ourselves to slow down, and taking time off to recreate and refresh. Humor, playfulness, being in the moment, and enjoying simple pleasures can help us bring joy back into our lives.

1. What gives you joy?
2. What is one thing you can do today that makes you laugh or smile?
3. When are you not conscious of time pressure?
4. What can you do to feel this way more often?

# CHAPTER FOUR

# Taking Care of Your Midlife Body

If any thing is sacred the human body is sacred.
— Walt Whitman, "I Sing the Body Electric," 1855

Remember when you took for granted that your finely tuned body would perform well despite the stresses you put it under? In midlife, when we start to notice illness and the physical changes associated with age, we awake to the importance and power of the body and the effect that personal health practices have on how well it functions. Suddenly it dawns on us. When we learn to understand, accept, and take responsibility for our physical health, we benefit from a massive surge of untapped energy. We can become better lovers and better parents and better friends. But, most importantly, we can be stronger and more confident in our ability to control how we live and enjoy each day.

Participants in the Healthy Boomer Midlife Survey identified three general areas as top priorities for change in their physical health:

- losing weight and eating in a healthier way
- getting in better physical shape and having more stamina
- stopping addictive behaviors, particularly smoking and excessive drinking

As we discussed in the previous chapter, the biggest barriers to making changes in physical health practices were a lack of time and low energy levels. This chapter describes the boomers' struggle with making changes in their personal health practices and provides some complementary specific strategies for successful change.

## SOME HIGHLIGHTS FROM THE HEALTHY
## BOOMER MIDLIFE SURVEY

---

### *Healthy Eating*
*How often do you eat three well-balanced meals each day?*

| | |
|---|---|
| Five to seven days per week | 47% |
| One to four days per week | 36% |
| No days per week | 16% |
| No answer | 1% |

---

*Does stress at work or in your personal relationships affect how you eat?*

| | |
|---|---|
| Yes | 56% |
| No | 44% |

---

### *Active Living*
*Is an active lifestyle/exercise important to you?*

| | |
|---|---|
| Yes | 87% |
| No | 9% |
| No answer | 4% |

---

*Do you think you get enough exercise to be healthy?*

| | |
|---|---|
| Yes | 33% |
| No | 51% |
| Do not know | 16% |

---

## Changes Worth Making

We were not surprised that weight loss was the number-one desired physical change in midlife. As the Big Generation has aged, weight problems, obesity, and related diseases such as diabetes, have increased substantially in North America. In addition to the health risks associated with being overweight, fat and weight gain are key issues in changes in our appearance that often accompany aging. Weight management is discussed in the next chapter. Here, we deal with the two lifestyle behaviors that most influence weight management – eating and physical activity. Efforts to lose weight need to focus on changing these two aspects of our lives, more than on the actual loss of weight. When we adopt healthy eating habits and regular physical activity patterns, weight control should naturally follow.

*Healthy Eating*

Busy people have a hard time practicing healthy eating. Even in our highly educated sample, fewer than half of our respondents said that they ate three well-balanced meals a day. "I need to develop the willpower to discipline myself and eat three balanced meals every day," said one man. A midlife woman said, "I want to eat regular meals and a minimum number of snacks, without overeating." Others talked about a desire to reduce the amount of high-calorie and high-fat foods they consumed. "I want to eliminate late-night snacks and eat salad for lunch instead of two sandwiches," said one man. Others talked about cutting down on sweets, fats, and starches, and of eating less of specific foods, such as chocolate.

Just slightly more than half of our respondents acknowledged that stress at home and at work affects how they eat – for the worse. "I have all kind of good intentions," said one woman, "but when things don't go right at the office, I reach for a strong coffee and a doughnut."

Many talked about how the time crunch and their fatigue interfered with their attempts to eat well. One woman said it this way: "By the time I get everyone else off, I just don't have time to have breakfast before I leave in the morning, so I snack at my desk. Sometimes I miss lunch as well. When I get home in the evening, I am so exhausted the last thing I want to do is cook a healthy meal from scratch. Take-out pizza seems like the best solution."

The tendency for North Americans to eat "on the run" is culturally sanctioned by our work habits and the preponderance of fast-food take-out businesses. Visitors from Europe and other countries comment on how we eat at our desks, in our cars, and on the street. Such behavior would be unacceptable in France or Greece, where sitting down to a complete meal is considered a sacred part of the day. Not surprisingly, the incidence of obesity and overweight is much higher in North America than it is in Europe. Fatigue and irregular eating patterns go hand in hand with the difficulty North Americans have in honoring a short break to enjoy their food.

*Active Living*

Although the respondents to our survey were more active than boomers as a whole, most believed that they needed more physical activity to be healthy. Their motivations for wanting to increase their levels of physical activity were varied:

- "I want to increase my physical stamina" (the most common answer).
- "I need more flexibility in my body, to lose weight, and to tune up my body."
- "I want to puff less when I climb stairs."
- "I want to be able to enjoy the sports I love."
- "My bone density is low, and I know that weight-bearing exercise and weight training will help."
- "I want to get in shape so I can go on a cycling trip to Vermont with my friends."
- "I want to find more time to be active with my kids – to go skating and swimming with them."
- "I think that increasing my activity levels would help me cope with stresses at work."
- "I have heard that men who are physically active are more active sexually. It makes sense – if you have energy for life, you have energy for intimacy."

We talked with Russ Kisby, former president of ParticipACTION, about how boomers see lack of time as the biggest barrier – and excuse – for not being more physically active. "There is good news for busy people in the research that has come out in the last few years," he says. "We have learned that even modest amounts of activity can have significant health benefits. As a bonus, we now know that you can obtain these health benefits by accumulating even thirty minutes of physical activity in three ten-minute segments throughout your day. This fact makes it hard to use 'no time' as an excuse."

Recently, Dr. JoAnn Manson, chief of Preventive Medicine at Harvard's Brigham and Women's Hospital, stated, "Regular physical activity is probably as close to a 'magic bullet' as we will come in modern medicine. If everyone were to walk briskly thirty minutes a day, we could cut the incidence of many chronic diseases by 30 to 40 per cent."

### Substance Misuse and Abuse

In Canada, some 25 per cent of men and 21 per cent of women aged thirty-five to sixty-five are smokers. They also tend to be the heaviest smokers – an average number of 21 cigarettes a day by men and 18 a day by women. In other words, midlife boomers who have not been able to quit smoking at this point are likely to be heavily addicted to nicotine.

Although we did not ask specifically about marijuana use, we know from our clinic that the boomer generation's appetite for recreational drugs has not vanished completely. However, the reasons for using these drugs have changed in many cases. Whereas the hip generation used recreational drugs to "expand their minds," people told us that they now use marijuana to treat themselves for "down" moods and to escape stress. Ironically, when used regularly, marijuana exacerbates feelings of lethargy and down moods. Others talked about cross-addictions. One fifty-four-year-old man said, "My smoking was associated with cocaine addiction. I only managed to get off cigarettes after I stopped using cocaine."

In adolescence and early adulthood, most of us believe that we are invincible. In midlife, fears about illness and death become real for smokers. "I quit after watching my father die a painful death from lung cancer," said one woman. "Thinking about my dad gave me lots of determination." A sixty-three-year-old woman told us that she had been trying to quit ever since her sister, who smoked three packs a day, died of respiratory failure at age fifty-two. "I succeeded on my third attempt with the help of a Zyban prescription and counseling from my family physician. I will never smoke again and I am working on my thirty-five-year-old daughter to get her to quit as well."

Many boomers told us that a few beers or glasses of good wine had become the reward they felt entitled to have after working hard all day. Unfortunately for some, this practice is a slippery slope towards alcohol misuse and abuse. "I kept telling myself I was a 'social drinker,' when in reality I was drinking almost a bottle of wine every night," said one woman. "I had developed a dependency, and I couldn't admit it to myself."

One forty-five-year-old woman told us how she and her husband began to drink as a way of coping with grief. "After our son died, my husband and I developed the habit of having a few drinks when we got home from work each day. We wore public faces all day, and came home to try to deal with how we really felt. The numbing effect of a stiff Black Russian really helped. After two years of this we realized we had a problem, and it was time to cope without the alcohol. It wasn't easy, but at this point we have cut back to occasional drinks on anniversary dates."

While most smokers acknowledged that abstinence was the only solution, when it came to alcohol the question of cutting down or cutting out completely was a much greater dilemma. Some respondents in the contemplation stage talked about their inability to make a decision because the cons did not yet outweigh the pros. "Sure, I would lose weight and have more energy in the evening if I stopped drinking," said one man, "but I like the taste; it relaxes me. I am never hung over, and it does not affect other people. In fact I would really miss having a few beers with friends on Fridays after work." Some try on a daily or intermittent basis to control their drinking. One man said, "I have conversations with myself every day about my drinking. I make a decision for that day. I can usually find other things I want to do, like spending time with the kids or going for a workout." One fifty-two-year-old woman said, "My mother is an alcoholic and I am constantly aware of the pull towards addiction. I have stopped drinking several times, and those times were affirming and liberating. It was a relief to know that I could do it."

Many people struggle with addictive behaviors for months and years. Sometimes, family members and intimate partners end up frustrated when an addicted person is not ready or willing to get treatment, or treatment is not helping. Some people can change addictive behaviors without professional assistance by moving through the stages of self-change described in Chapter 2. For some, programs like Alcoholics Anonymous or Women for Sobriety provide the support they need. Others opt for individual counseling, special programs in their communities, residential treatments, or a combination of approaches. In these cases, treatment initiatives work best when they complement and build on the Stages of Change process.

SOME HIGHLIGHTS FROM THE HEALTHY
BOOMER MIDLIFE SURVEY

### Tobacco
*Have you smoked cigarettes at any time in your life?*

| | |
|---|---|
| Never smoked | 49% |
| Quit smoking | 36% |
| Smoke cigarettes now | 15% |

### Alcohol
*Do you drink alcohol?*

| | |
|---|---|
| Daily | 14% |
| Occasionally | 60% |
| Not at all | 24% |
| No answer | 2% |

*How many drinks do you have in an average week?*
*(1 drink = 1 glass of wine, 1 oz spirit, 1 beer)*

| | |
|---|---|
| 1 to 5 drinks | 45% |
| 5 to 15 drinks | 22% |
| More than 20 drinks | 3% |
| No answer or not applicable | 30% |

*Has anyone expressed concern about your drinking in the past five years?*

| | |
|---|---|
| No | 69% |
| Yes | 7% |
| Not applicable | 24% |

*Do you ever drink as a result of stress in your work life or in your relationships?*

| | |
|---|---|
| No | 71% |
| Yes | 5% |
| Not applicable | 24% |

*Have you ever stopped drinking completely or deliberately cut back*
*on the amount you drink, at any point in your life?*

| | |
|---|---|
| Cut back on drinking | 11% |
| Stopped drinking completely | 22% |
| Neither | 42% |
| Not applicable | 25% |

## Helpful Strategies

Successful change takes place in a series of well-defined steps, as discussed in Chapter 2. For people in midlife, strategies to overcome the perceived barriers of limited time and energy are especially important (see Chapter 3). Here we present some specific ideas that seem to be especially important when it comes to you and your physical health.

### 1. Strive for Moderation

As discussed in Chapter 2 on the Stages of Change and Chapter 5 on weight control, realistic goal-setting is critical to success. For example, it is far more realistic to start walking for twenty minutes three times a week on your way home from the bus stop than to tell yourself that you will immediately walk all the way to work and back, and join a soccer team, and start jogging again.

The other danger in trying to perform at the highest levels is now referred to on the Internet as "extreme self-care." When we looked for websites that used this phrase, we found thousands of hits. Many of them advertised products (such as high-performance drinks) and services (such as professional trainers) that aim to help you reach the ultimate in physical fitness, weight control, and other such goals. Most of us know someone who has become obsessed with health, fitness, or nutrition to the point at which it becomes counterproductive, and even harmful. "My obsession with running on hard pavement and over-training for marathons led to a number of injuries that have now made running impossible for me," said one man.

Dr. Steven Bratman, a physician and self-professed recovering health nut, has written a book on the symptoms and treatment of an obsession with food quality, *Health Food Junkies* (2000). While "orthorexia nervosa" is not yet classified as an official psychological disorder, it is increasingly talked about in health circles. According to Bratman, orthorexics fear that food is unsafe and they spend inordinate amounts of time and energy searching for "pure" and "natural" foods. As a result, their diets are often very restricted and may be low in protein, vitamins, minerals, and fat.

One woman talked about her obsession with getting enough of all the vitamins, minerals, and other nutrients she thought she needed to be healthy and ward off the aches, colds, and health problems she was afraid of getting. "I was spending a fortune in supplements," she said. "I was embarrassed to show a dietitian all of the pills and drinks that I was taking. She pointed out to me that some nutrients could not be accessed by the body in pill form, and that often I was just peeing out excess nutrients I could not absorb. With her help, I have learned to be less extreme. I also realized that what I really need to do is take the time to prepare and enjoy fresh foods, instead of trying to find health in a pill bottle."

## 2. Seek Support

One man in our clinic had been trying to quit smoking for many years. Each time he came in, Dr. Lhotsky discussed quitting with him, because of a variety of medical problems that were linked to his use of tobacco. Finally, she told him, "Don't worry. This time I will not give you the 'motivational talk' about quitting smoking." He was stunned and got very upset. "How dare you give up on me!" he yelled. Then he relaxed and explained that he had in fact finally managed to quit. He had been waiting to hear her spiel so that he could surprise her with the good news.

Your family physician can be a powerful support, as can nurses, psychotherapists, addiction counselors, and other professionals who work in community programs. However, most often our family members and friends help us make and maintain changes.

When it comes to increasing physical activity levels, Russ Kisby says, "Over three decades of working with ParticipACTION, one of my major conclusions is the power of 'the buddy system.' Most people decide at some point that it would be desirable to get more exercise. So off they go – with enthusiasm and the best of intentions – for one or two days. Only a small percentage find they are able to maintain their initial commitment on their own! However, people who seek out a friend who shares their goal to be active tend to have substantially greater success in sticking with it. We all have days when we just don't feel like it, or perceive we are too busy. There is nothing like a buddy to cajole us into taking action, while also making the activity experience more enjoyable."

Three siblings told us how they used a technique called "contracting" to support each other in a mutual decision to quit smoking. One of the sisters said, "We all decided to quit, mostly for my brother, who was the heaviest smoker and had asthma and frequent chest infections. We made a deal. We all put down money – a large enough sum for each of us to feel it. To be sure we were going to be even more motivated, we agreed that those who started again would have to reveal 'a big family secret' about themselves." The two sisters were successful in becoming and remaining non-smokers. "Unfortunately my brother did not last," explains one of the sisters. "But we have not given up on him. He has promised that he will try again in a few months and we are helping him get ready for that."

Three businesswomen in their fifties started out using money as an incentive to lose weight and ended up using it to cement their friendship and commitment to changing the way they lived. One of them explained: "We got the idea because our husbands had successfully lost weight with a $250 bet on who could lose it first. They all lost weight, and the one that got to his goal first won the money. We each put in $2,000 – the amount that we would have spent going to a commercial weight-loss clinic." They agreed that the winner would use the money to travel to a luxurious spa.

Over the next few months they were there for each other – exercising together and giving each other lots of support over the phone. In the end, all three achieved their desired weight. "Rather than reward the person who got there first, we decided to celebrate our friendship and success together. We used the money we had put in the pot to go to Vancouver to attend one of our daughters' weddings and live it up. We were three svelte and happy ladies!"

*3. Debunk the Myth "It Just Takes Willpower."*
"It's my own laziness and lack of self-discipline."
   "It is easier to sit here than go out for a walk or run."

"I just need to pull up my socks and do it."

"I'm ashamed of my lack of willpower."

When it comes to getting active, losing weight, and changing eating patterns, we heard these kinds of self-blaming remarks over and over. But people who rely solely on willpower set themselves up for failure. Would you advise someone else to kick themselves when they were down? It takes commitment and solid preparation to overcome that old reptilian brain's resistance to change. When you take concrete steps to make the healthy choices the easy choices, you increase your confidence that you will succeed. This in turn increases your chances of success.

### 4. Build a Supportive Environment Around You

Our environment has a strong influence on how we behave. For example, there is little doubt that changes in public attitudes toward secondhand smoke, combined with laws requiring smoke-free buildings, have significantly influenced smoking rates in the last twenty years. One woman said, "At first I was really pissed off when my employer announced we were going smoke-free. But then I realized, 'Hey, I have been wanting to cut down or even quit. I can use this as an opportunity to help me do so.'" Similarly, it is a lot easier to make healthful food choices when your work cafeteria offers fresh, attractive salads and skim milk, rather than just burgers, fries, and pop. "When I got serious about eating better, I went on a walkabout to find healthy eating places near my work," said one woman. "Then I convinced a friend to walk there with me twice a week and brought my lunch on the other days."

Numerous people told us how they successfully used a new or changed physical environment as an impetus to change their behavior. One couple quit smoking when they moved into a new house; another family outlawed eating on the run in their new car. One woman told us how she used a trip to Europe, where she would be staying with non-smoking in-laws for a month, as her chance to quit smoking. She went public with her decision before she left and as soon as she arrived. Because she had also prepared herself for handling her old environment when she returned, she was able to maintain her lifestyle change. Another man told us how he and a group of colleagues successfully lobbied their employer to put in showers, a change room, and a place for bicycle storage when they were renovating one of the company's buildings. "It just makes it so much easier to bike to work or to go for a jog at lunch," he says. "Even the VP uses it."

In terms of influencing behavior change, the social environment can be even more powerful than the physical one. One hopes that family members, friends, and colleagues will support positive changes (as discussed above). Unfortunately, this is not always the case. For example, many alcoholics need to restructure their social lives, so that they can get away from drinking buddies who support their alcohol abuse rather than their sobriety. "I had to change who I hung out with," said one man. "Alcoholics Anonymous helps – it offers me alcohol-free social interactions and support. I go to meetings when I am traveling on business as well. I meet others who are staying sober and I have no excuse to wander into a bar to find some conversation."

The media have always had a strong influence on boomers' behaviors. Many smokers who have successfully quit now see that the tobacco industry's marketing tactics were part of the reason they started to smoke in the first place. Now, they are even more enraged about industry advertising, particularly that which is directed at their daughters. "My daughter is convinced that smoking will keep her slim," says one woman. "No wonder. Virginia Slims is the world's bestselling cigarette to women. Think about it – the name of the cigarette describes what young women want to be!"

Sometimes, media personalities can positively influence people making lifestyle choices, as in the case of the late journalist and broadcaster, Peter Gzowski. Many boomers regarded Gzowski as a friend they knew from listening to him every day on CBC Radio's *Morningside* program. Ironically, he died during National Non-Smoking Week in January 2002, of chronic obstructive pulmonary disease, despite kicking his three-pack-a-day habit in 1999. Many believe that he provided a powerful incentive for other smokers. His thoughts on quitting were published in a 2001 essay, entitled "How to Quit Smoking in 50 Years or Less," which appeared in the book *Addicted: Notes from the Belly of the Beast* (Douglas & McIntyre). At the time of his death, one caller to a smokers' helpline said that having heard Gzowski talk about quitting and the tributes to him after his death made him call to get help.

**From the Research**

*Gender Differences in Self-Care Practices*

According to the Canadian 1998/99 National Population Health Survey, men and women differ in the ways they care for their own health.

Nutrition tends to be more important to women. Women were more likely than men to consider overall health, weight, and specific diseases when choosing food. Men, however, were more likely than women to engage in vigorous activity during their leisure time. Yet, despite this, 42 per cent of men were overweight, compared with 24 per cent of women.

From age twenty-five on, a higher proportion of men than women smoked daily. Men are far more likely than women to "binge drink," defined as consuming at least five alcoholic drinks at one sitting.

Women are more likely than men to experience stress. They use health-care services more than men do – both mainstream medicine and complementary services such as acupuncturists, massage therapists, and naturopaths. Women also use over-the-counter or prescription medication more than men do. Fully 71 per cent of women said they had used pain relievers in the month before the survey, compared with 58 per cent of men. This may be related to the greater prevalence of conditions such as arthritis and migraine among women.

Source: Statistics Canada, Health Statistics Division. "The Health Divide: How the Sexes Differ," *Health Reports*, Vol. 12, No. 3 (2001).

**On the Lighter Side**

*Healthy Living for a Long Time*

A middle-aged man goes to the doctor and says: "Doc, I would like to live a very long time. What should I do?"

"I think that is a wise decision," the doctor replies. "Let's see, do you smoke?"

"Yes, half a pack a day."

"Well, starting *right now*, there's no more smoking." The man agrees. The doctor then asks, "Do you drink?"

"Oh, well, Doc, not much, just a bit of wine with my meals, and a beer or two every once in a while."

"Starting now, you drink only water. No exceptions." The man is a bit upset, but again agrees. Then the doctor asks, "How do you eat?"

"Oh, gee, you know, Doc, normal stuff like meat, rice, and potatoes."

"Starting now you are going on a very strict diet. You are going to eat only raw vegetables, with no dressing, and non-fat cottage cheese."

The man is now really worried and says, "Doc, is all this really necessary?"

"Do you want to live a very long time?"

"Well, yes, but. . . ."

"No buts about it, then! It's absolutely necessary. And don't even think of breaking that diet." Now the man is quite restless, but the doctor continues. "Do you ever have sex?"

"Yeah, once a week or so . . . but only with my wife!" he adds hurriedly.

"As soon as you get out of here, you are going to buy twin beds. No more sex for you! Absolutely none."

The man is now scared and downright appalled. "Doc . . . Are you sure that I'm going to live longer this way?"

"Well, I can't guarantee it, but however long you live I assure you that at least it's going to *seem* like an eternity!"

## Questions to Reflect On

Making a change in your physical health practices means setting realistic goals, preparing for change, and building a supportive environment more than exerting willpower. Change is not easy, but it can be done.

1. What one area of your physical health would you like to change?
2. How can you realistically influence your physical and social environments so that they support your decision to change?
3. How else can you prepare to make that change? Be as specific as you can.

# CHAPTER FIVE

# *Mirror, Mirror . . .*

Mirror, mirror on the wall, who's the fairest one of all?
— The Wicked Queen in *Snow White*, 1938

Somewhere between the ages of forty and fifty, we look in the mirror and are shocked at what we see reflected back. We flinch at the sight of wrinkles, double chins, or gray hair. We ask ourselves, "What happened?" "Is that person really me?" "When did I get old?" As one boomer in our survey put it: "One day I saw a matronly woman looking back from the mirror, and I realized it was me."

Whether we are male or female, physical appearance has always been important to us. As infants, we were adored because of the way we looked. As teenagers, appearance was linked to popularity and potential love relationships. As young adults, physical attractiveness affected how we went about finding a mate and making friends. Now, at midlife, personal appearance takes a new and special spin. No matter how many friends tell us we look the same, the reality is hard to deny. We are getting older, and it shows – in the mirror and on the tennis court. Gone are the days when we could stay out late, drink a lot, and still perform effortlessly at sports the next day.

We try to rationalize our fears about aging and the changes in how we look. After all, we have years of experience and accomplishments. We have developed important relationships and unique personalities. We are raising families and making important contributions to our communities and our occupations. How we look is trivial when compared to these accomplishments. We should be able to put these concerns aside, right?

Wrong.

Yes, these accomplishments are more important than how we look. But as a society we remain obsessed with youth and beauty. We hold a lot of stereotypes and negative images about aging that get in the way of our accepting changes in how we look. As individuals, we long for one more chance to be adored for our appearance. Maybe, if we became the fairest again, we would find unconditional love and happiness. And as we watch age creep up on us, we are consciously or unconsciously worried about the link between aging and death – a reality that the boomer generation desperately denies.

In this chapter we look at boomers' attitudes and experiences related to physical appearance. Our survey respondents were candid. It troubles them that they are no longer "the fairest of them all." But at the same time, they recognize and appreciate the gains of growing older. In the end, their message stresses the need to find the middle road, by practicing self-care activities that keep you healthy and feeling young. But they must be tempered with a reality check. Our looks are changing. We'd better accept it . . . and get on with life.

### When Was the First Time You Felt Middle-Aged?

We asked our survey respondents, "When was the first time you felt middle-aged?" All of us can relate to some of the wise – and often funny – answers to this question.

For many midlife men and women, reactions from younger people – especially salesclerks, gas attendants, and teenagers – triggered the first feelings of being middle-aged. One man said, "When all the young salesclerks started call me 'Sir,' I knew I had hit middle age." Ironically, for another man, it was a compliment from a young lady who said, "You're in pretty good shape for a guy your age."

Several people referred to the first time they looked in the mirror and saw how much they now resembled their mothers or fathers. "Our culture worships youth," said one woman, "and being young and attractive was part of my identity. Suddenly that has changed and I look like my mother. That is not a bad thing – my mom is very attractive. But it is hard to be moved into her age category." Another woman in her fifties described a traumatic moment of revelation. "What a shock! I was visiting my dad's retirement home and someone asked me if I was a resident!"

Many women spoke about feeling "invisible" in middle age. One fifty-five-year-old woman said, "Men no longer give me the eye when I walk into a room. When men speak to me, they look through me rather than at me."

Another woman described her discomfort at her husband's Christmas party. "The median age in his company is early thirties. I felt completely invisible, uninteresting, and irrelevant to most of the people there." Several women expressed anger and frustration that societal views of midlife women are so dismissive. "There is such a passion for youth in our culture that society treats middle-aged women as invisible. Wisdom and experience seem to count for men, but not for women."

Significant birthdays and having to write down one's age on a form are other triggers for feeling middle-aged. One man said, "Now, on questionnaires and surveys I am ticking off the age group to the right of the page. Years ago it was to the left." One woman described why she left town on her fortieth birthday. "I couldn't face a surprise party with all those jokes about being over the hill. I didn't want to be forty. I didn't want a party, but I also didn't want to stay home and watch television and wait for the phone to ring. I just wanted to get out of town." Another woman described how her fortieth birthday turned into a celebration of her courage and her future. "I am deathly afraid of heights, but I was visiting Australia and made up my mind I was going to climb Ayers Rock on my birthday. I made it to the top feeling exhilarated and a little panicky. My heart was pounding in my chest. I wrote my name in the book they have there, and added 'born forty years ago today.' The man behind me read it out loud to all the other climbers, and everyone applauded. I looked down from that magical, mystical place and I felt alive, blessed, and ready for the next ten years."

For others, becoming a grandparent was a clear signal that midlife had begun in earnest. Most explained that it was the lead-up, not the event itself, that made them feel anxious. One woman explained it this way: "The thought of my children having children made me feel old. When my daughter got pregnant, I was excited but depressed. I wasn't ready to be a 'granny' and all that meant in the traditional sense. Once the baby was born, I was ecstatic. I adore him. I am proud to tell everyone that I am a grandmother . . . and I especially love it when I babysit and people think that he is mine!"

An increasing number of boomers are becoming parents of young children in midlife. One fifty-one-year-old woman said, "Being a midlife mom of young children is a blessing in many ways, but I also worry about being around for them when they are young adults. When I think of how old I'll be when they are ten and fifteen, I get very conscious of my appearance. I don't want to be mistaken for their grandmother. I think I'm much more concerned about looking old than I would be if I didn't have young kids."

### SOME HIGHLIGHTS FROM THE HEALTHY
### BOOMER MIDLIFE SURVEY

*Noticeable changes in physical appearance over the last ten years*

|  | Women | Men |
|---|---|---|
| Graying hair | 73% | 87% |
| Hair loss | 13% | 40% |
| Increased facial hair (women) | 45% | NA |
| Weight gain | 70% | 47% |
| Weight loss | 9% | 0% |
| Wrinkles and changes in skin tone | 65% | 23% |
| Decreased muscle tone | 40% | 43% |
| Glasses or bifocals | 64% | 40% |
| Dental problems | 25% | 40% |
| Varicose veins | 23% | 0% |
| Bunions | 20% | 0% |
| Looking more confident | 27% | 20% |

*Accepting of changes in physical appearance*

|  | Women | Men |
|---|---|---|
| Accepting | 43% | 53% |
| Somewhat accepting | 41% | 33% |
| Neither accepting nor unaccepting | 5% | 14% |
| Somewhat unaccepting | 11% | 0% |
| Unaccepting | 0% | 0% |

| *Is there a male menopause?* | Women | Men |
| --- | --- | --- |
| Yes | 65% | 40% |
| No | 8% | 18% |
| Do not know | 27% | 42% |

## Grieving the Loss of Youthful Looks

For both men and women, graying hair, weight gain, wrinkles and changes in skin tone, and the need to wear glasses or bifocals were the most common changes in appearance associated with aging. Women were three times as likely as men to have noticed wrinkles and changes in their skin tone. They were more likely to have bunions – no doubt as a result of wearing pointy or overly tight shoes – and varicose veins – sometimes as a result of pregnancies. On the other hand, the men in our survey (40%) were more likely to have experienced dental problems than the women were (25%). This may reflect findings that women visit the dentist for preventive reasons more regularly and faithfully than men. Men are more likely to visit the dentist only when they have problems.

Of all of the changes that accompany aging, wearing glasses seemed most acceptable to midlife boomers. This may be at least partly because wearing attractive lenses is now acceptable for all ages in our culture. "I used to need to wear glasses," said one woman. "Now I *have* to wear them. My arms just aren't long enough when I try to read the paper." One woman talked enthusiastically about getting laser surgery to correct her vision problems. "It was wonderful. I went without glasses for eight years, but now I need them again for reading. I have accepted it. I hang them around my neck. It reminds me of my mom or of an old schoolmarm, but it really is the most practical thing to do. Otherwise I put them down and lose them."

Social pressures to look youthful and attractive figure large in how we perceive the changes in our appearance. For men, the decrease in muscle tone was a foremost concern, reflecting society's emphasis on the importance of a strong, virile, and muscular physique for men. "I hate my pot," said one man, "but it is really hard to get rid of it. I look around at middle-aged guys who have even bigger bellies than mine and I think, 'Man, that is gross.' I have to do something about it." A related concern for men is the loss of fitness and strength that accompanies aging. "Now my back gives me trouble when I lift heavy things," said one man. "I know it is related to the weight gain around my middle and the lack of strength in my back." Another man remarked, "My son beats me every time in one-on-one basketball now. That hurts, because I was pretty good in my day. It makes me feel old."

One man told a story about peeing in the bush beside his nine-year-old grandson. "Here I was with my pee kind of dribbling down, while he shot his up and out towards the distance. I knew then that I was definitely getting older."

Not surprisingly, women talked more about the need to remain youthful, beautiful, and slim. "I hate it that my clothes don't fit around my stomach any more," said one woman. Another remarked, "As a formerly fit, attractive, and young-looking person, I find it difficult to equate who I am with who I used to be. It seriously affects my ability to enjoy how I look and feel, and to see myself as sexy or good-looking."

While most of our respondents were trying to lose weight, we see numerous boomer women in our clinic who are obsessed with maintaining an unhealthy, very low weight through near-starvation levels of eating and excessive exercise. One of these women told us, "I finally said enough is enough. What good is being ultra-slim if you ruin your health and quality of life in the process?"

Ironically, at this stage of life, men and women have different problems with hair. While men bemoan the loss of hair, and its migration from the top of the head to the ears and nose, women are horrified by the sudden appearance of chin hairs and other facial fuzz, while the hair on the tops of their heads becomes thinner.

On the positive side, 27 per cent of women and 20 per cent of men said that they looked more confident. In their written comments, numerous women said that they liked themselves better now than they did when they were young and constantly filled with angst about how they looked compared with others. "I like myself now," said one woman. "I find myself attractive . . . I am strong and well built – not thin – but I have a presence."

### Strategies for Dealing with Midlife Changes in Appearance

In our survey, the majority of respondents said they were "accepting" – 53 per cent of men and 43 per cent of women – or "somewhat accepting" – 33 per cent of men and 41 per cent of women – of midlife changes in their appearance. Some 11 per cent of women were "somewhat unaccepting" of the changes. One woman said, "I always look tired. I am definitely not very accepting of the changes in my appearance. If I had the money, I would have my eyes done and my face lifted."

This does not mean that people were "letting themselves go" and making no effort to maintain their bodies, their health, and their looks. On the contrary, both women and men were making efforts to lose weight, get in shape, wear attractive clothes, and look after their eyes, teeth, hair, and skin. Here are some of the things that helped survey participants deal with the physical changes they had experienced in the last ten years.

#### Loving Partners and Supportive Friends

More than anything else, respondents said that reassurance and sexy looks from their intimate partners were the most helpful factor in feeling good about how they looked. One woman said, "I have a loving partner who still looks at me in that certain way." Another said, "My partner still adores me, and always tells me how he loves me and my body."

Some people referred to comfort in the company of others. "It really helps to have friends going through the same thing," said one man. Several women referred to the importance of support from their women friends. "We commiserate about our expanded waistlines and liver-spotted hands. My best friend and I often shop together, and it helps to have her view on which styles of clothes suit me since I have gained fifteen pounds. We support each other in our choice to never wear those pointy shoes with high heels again."

#### Finding Humor in It All

"You have to laugh about it sometimes," said one woman. "My women friends and I joke about our chin hairs. I thought it was hilarious when Rosie O'Donnell grew hers on television and then actually showed up with them beaded!"

Midlife changes in appearance and our denial of aging have become popular subjects for writers and journalists who are in midlife themselves. Humorist Anne Hines told us that having fun with our ambivalent feelings about aging makes for great copy that a lot of people can appreciate. In an article in *Chatelaine* magazine in January 1999 she addresses her denial of hitting middle age at age forty. "My hair is starting to gray, but that began around the time my daughter started picking out her own clothes. Awareness of my aging came with the realizations that I will buy anything from a salesperson who calls me 'Miss,' and that, if a construction worker whistles, it means there is a teenage girl behind me. I know I can't stop the march of time; I just wish it wasn't using my face as the main parade route."

Bill Giurato, a forty-four-year-old man from Burnaby, British Columbia, wrote in the Toronto *Globe and Mail* on March 11, 2002, about coming to terms with his midlife bushy eyebrows. He resorted to scissors, hair gel, and tweezers at the hand of his merciless wife, but stopped short of waxing and electrolysis. He despaired that such a crisis could be brought about "by something as petty as unregenerate eyebrows." In the end, he decided to admit defeat. "If not young in appearance," he wrote, "at least I am intelligent enough to know that some battles are better unfought; some hairs are better left unplucked."

*Appreciating the Gains That Aging Brings*

While respondents in our survey readily identified how uncomfortable they feel about looking older, they also described some major positive transformations in how they felt about themselves. Here is what four women said:

- "I am more confident about who I am. For a long time I worried about appearance, but not now."
- "I cannot compete with those twenty-two-year-olds out there! This is somewhat of a relief. I am glad to get beyond petty vanity and enjoy my newfound confidence. I am now invisible to men, and this is liberating. I can concentrate on doing the things I want to do."
- "I want to grow old proud of the wisdom I have gained and not just focused on the outer package. I resent the marketing of anti-age

beauty products. My mother is eighty-one and she is beautiful. It is the eyes and the smile that count, not how young your skin looks."

- "The face of my youth may be gone, but so is the girl who agonized every day about how that face looked. I like the view I carry of myself inside now, and I reach out to others because I am less concerned about how I look. It's a good feeling."

Others talked about how the mental, emotional, and spiritual gains of aging offset changes in their appearance. One man said, "With aging has come my spiritual growth and the benefits of life experience and wisdom. I am happier now than I have ever been."

### Active Healthy Living

Almost all those who responded to our survey talked about their efforts to exercise, improve their diets, and lose weight as ways to look and feel better. "I weigh ten pounds more than when I was younger," said one man, "but I figure if I stay active and fit, I will still look good. More importantly, it gives me the energy I need to do all the things I want to do each day." One woman noted that she was glad she had stopped smoking in her early thirties. "When I look at the faces, teeth, and fingers of my friends that smoke, they look so much older."

Maintaining an active, healthy way of life in the middle years is not easy. Some of the barriers – and ideas for overcoming them – are discussed in Chapters 2 and 3, and later in this chapter, in "A Weighty Matter." The important point is that boomers know that practicing healthy lifestyles is critical to looking and feeling better.

### Shifting Your Focus

Germaine Greer writes in her book *The Change* (1992) that it is only when women end the fretful struggle to be beautiful that they can turn their gaze outward and feast on what is beautiful around them. Instead of worrying so much about how we appear to others, we need to get back inside our own skins and nourish ourselves by surrounding ourselves with beauty. One fifty-three-year-old woman said, "I am trying hard to be less concerned about the signs of aging on my face. When I forget about it, I have more energy to enjoy the beauty of nature. Then I feel more relaxed and probably look better anyway!" If we continue to compare ourselves to others – "I look at other women who are my age, and I think I look pretty good" – we keep our focus on outward appearance. Ultimately, we will feel that inner glow when we are fulfilled, immersed in life, and affirming our own unique attractiveness and value.

### Positive Self-Care

Most of the respondents in our survey said that it is important to make efforts to look your best at any age. At the same time, the women we spoke with were often almost apologetic about caring for themselves, as if doing so implied vanity or selfishness. One said, "I try to dress well and look after myself so that I will age gracefully. It's not just vanity. Feeling well emotionally and in control of my health is most important to me. When I am in control, I look and act more confident and attractive."

Several people talked about how they now pay more attention to their oral and dental health, especially since midlife gum problems can lead to pain and costly dental bills. "My dentist suggested I invest in a good electric toothbrush and use it regularly. I did. Now every time I go for a checkup, the hygienist says that my gum recession is getting better."

Several women told us that they now make regular foot care a part of their routine. One woman said, "I go for regular pedicures to get rid of calluses. My feet look great in sandals, and it is one of the best treats I can give myself. A good foot massage is one of the most relaxing and heavenly experiences I have ever had."

Most midlife women – and increasingly men in midlife – pay special attention to caring for their skin. The first stop is usually the cosmetics counter, where a staggering array of moisturizers and "anti-aging" creams is available. Moisturizers are important rejuvenators for aging skin for both women and men. Several women told us their husbands started to use their moisturizing creams after shaving, and now they are sold on them. One man said, "Why shouldn't we guys get the benefit and nice feeling that comes with using these products? I look and feel a lot better when the skin on my face is not all harsh and peeling off."

The more difficult choices come with the so-called anti-aging products, complete with aloe, vitamin C, vitamin E, and other ingredients that are "scientifically formulated" to make skin younger-looking. Over-the-counter creams containing alpha hydroxy acids (AHA) and vitamin C have been shown to be somewhat helpful; however, prices for a small jar range from $25 to $150. Prescription creams with greater strengths of an active ingredient such as topical tretinoin can reduce small facial lines and wrinkles, but can also cause mild to severe peeling and redness.

### Cosmetic Procedures, Surgical and Nonsurgical

More and more boomers – particularly women, but increasingly men as well – are choosing cosmetic surgery as a way to look younger and improve their self-image and appearance. Technological developments such as the use of lasers and endoscopic equipment have made these procedures safer and less invasive. New natural and synthetic filler materials provide more natural-looking results that appear less "operated on." (For example, a variety of solid and semi-solid materials as well as tissue flaps and collagen from your own skin are used to produce the trendy, full "hot lips" that Goldie Hawn displayed so well in the classic boomer chick flick *The First Wives Club*.)

Studies show that 97 per cent of facial-surgery patients are happy with their results. Of the few who report dissatisfaction, most say the procedure failed to meet their expectations. This emphasizes the importance of having realistic expectations. Cosmetic facial surgery can improve your appearance, but it is not a magic wand.

Nonsurgical cosmetic procedures, which are less expensive, faster, and less invasive than surgical procedures, now account for 79 per cent of all cosmetic procedures. The top five are chemical peels, microdermabrasion, sclerotherapy (treatment of aesthetically unacceptable veins, including varicose veins), Botox injection, and laser hair removal. Botox injections, for example, take from fifteen to forty-five minutes, and you can return to work the next day. Botox is injected to counteract the wrinkles, furrows, and grooves caused by active expression muscles in the forehead and around the eyes and nose. It paralyzes small areas of these muscles for three to nine months, which softens the lines and smoothes out wrinkles.

Writing in *Canadian Living* magazine in February 2002, staff member **Pauline Anderson** described her foray into this brave new world. Anderson, who was forty-eight years old and the mother of preteens when she wrote about her experience, is fit and thinks young. But when she looked in the mirror, "a blotched shrunken face stared back." Anderson, who had never been vain about her skin, reasoned, "I'm probably healthier and I have more energy now than when I was in my twenties. So why shouldn't I look as young as I feel?" Yet she admitted that she had mixed emotions, including guilt, curiosity, and skepticism, when she volunteered to test out five of the new procedures over twelve weeks for a total cost of $4,000. When it was over, almost everyone, including her twelve-year-old son, noticed that she looked better. And for Anderson, the most important result was learning a lesson she believes other women need to learn – "that you are allowed, sometimes, to do something nice for yourself."

### Saving Face

More than any other generation, the boomers have brought the issue of cosmetic surgery out of the closet. In January 2001, *National Post* columnist **Sondra Gotlieb** published a series of will she?/won't she? articles about having cosmetic surgery. She decided to go ahead and have a facelift. Then she wrote in great and often hilarious detail about the decision-making process, choosing the right surgeon, her husband Alan's reaction, and the whole painful ordeal. We spoke with Sondra about a year and a half after her surgery about her perspective on it now.

"The memory has faded," she says, "but I remember that it hurt a lot more than I thought it would. I'm still really glad I did it, even with all the pain. I used to hate looking in the mirror. I had a round, fat face and now I have a thinner face."

We asked if she thought women were more open about cosmetic surgery now than in the past. "No, people aren't, at least here in Canada. In the United States people are far more open. I know some women who have had facelifts and they won't admit it. People will say, 'You look good; I'm going to do it too,' even when they already have had the procedure done. Only three or four people said, 'I love it. I've had one too.'"

When we asked about her husband's reactions, she said that he was initially against it. Because Sondra has some serious health problems, Alan was opposed to any non-essential surgery. In addition, when Sondra showed him photos of women who had had facelifts, he didn't think they looked all that great. He couldn't see much difference in the Before and After. But now, Sondra says, Alan really likes the result. "He was amazed. He said, 'Oh my God, you've got a profile! You haven't had one in twenty years.'"

Sondra is not interested in undergoing further cosmetic procedures. "I don't want my eyes done. I don't want the pain. I'd never do Botox. It seems kind of stupid, going every four months. I know someone who has had three facelifts, and now she's doing Botox. After so many procedures, there's a certain look – a kind of an expressionless face; you can't tell what she is thinking. Now, I can look at my photographs without feeling sick. I've discovered that for some reason, I look better in hats. I'm done with surgery."

People who undergo cosmetic surgery often face moral judgments – How can I justify spending this kind of money on my vanity? There are fears – What if the surgery is botched? What if I look like the Bride of Frankenstein? How much pain will there be? Sometimes the most important questions don't get asked: Why am I really doing this? What am I trying to accomplish? What are my fantasies of how this will change my life? In the end, it's not so much about doing it or not doing it. It is about asking the right questions of yourself, as well as of your medical consultant.

**Susan**, a fifty-two-year-old teacher, describes why she got an eyelid lift and how it made it her feel. "Every time I looked in the mirror, it seemed like my eyelids were drooping more. I knew that it ran in the family. My mother, who is in her eighties, has just decided to have the same operation for medical reasons. Her eyelids droop so much that they interfere with her vision."

Susan admits that vanity was also, to some degree, a factor in her decision. "This caused me to reflect on my value system, to ask myself why appearance was important to me. I came to the conclusion that it is not wrong to want to look your best. Many people spend $600 on a new coat or far more on frivolous purchases. Why should I feel guilty about spending money on something permanent that would make me look and feel better? I had no illusions that the surgery would make me look like a spring chicken again. But I knew I did not want to end up with eyelids virtually covering my eyes . . . which my husband says are my best feature."

Susan chose an experienced surgeon who had practiced restorative surgery in a hospital before opening his own clinic in cosmetic surgery. "He was recommended to me personally by several people, and I had total confidence in his credentials and ability to do the job," says Susan. She had two consultations with him. At the first one, Susan stated her goals and reasons for wanting the surgery. The surgeon explained the procedure and explored the options with her. "The second consultation felt like it was more to reassure him than me," says Susan. "He wanted to be sure that I did not have unreasonable expectations of what the surgery would do and that I had no doubts about going ahead."

Susan opted for a local anaesthetic. The operation was painless and took about one hour. "I have to admit I was pretty shocked when I looked in the mirror the next day," she says. "My face was swollen and my eyes were black and blue. I looked pretty dreadful." Susan followed her surgeon's advice for recovery. Within three days the swelling had dissipated, and within two to three weeks all traces of the surgery were gone.

Four years later, Susan says that she is totally happy with her decision to have the surgery. "Because I had it done earlier rather than later, people were unaware that an eyelid lift was responsible for the changes in how I looked. They kept telling me that I looked 'rested' or 'healthy' or that my eyes were attractive. I don't look younger, but I look better for the age I am. I have no hesitation in saying that it was the best $600 I ever spent!"

What advice does Susan offer to other boomers who are considering cosmetic surgery? "First," she says, "you need to research your surgeon's credentials. Choose an experienced doctor whom you trust, preferably one that has had experience in restorative plastic surgery as well as cosmetic surgery. Never go into debt to finance the procedure. If you can't save up the money ahead of time, it is too expensive to do. Lastly, be realistic about what the procedure will do. Cosmetic surgery is not going to get you a new job or transform your relationships. It can make you feel happier about your appearance, and that is a good thing."

If you are considering cosmetic procedures, consider the following points:

- Do your research very well, both about the procedure itself and about the health professional or surgeon who will perform it.
- It makes sense to use the least-invasive procedures to accomplish your aim – less downtime after, less pain, and less expense.

- Think of yourself as a unique, priceless work of art. Now, with the patina of age showing, there are no others like you. Weigh very carefully the pros and cons of restoration efforts.
- Take an honest look at any "hidden agendas" you may have – for example, believing that your life will be different, or that you won't feel as depressed if you have this procedure.

**Great Ways to Improve Your Smile**

In our interviews with boomers who read our first book, several people suggested that we should have talked about oral health in midlife and particularly about procedures for protecting our gums and brightening our smiles. Here, with the assistance of Dr. Andrea Veisman, who maintains a family and cosmetic dentistry practice in Toronto, is some of the latest information and best advice.

"The desire for a whiter, brighter smile is among the top dental concerns I hear from my midlife patients," says Dr. Veisman. Current methods for whitening the teeth include bleaching, veneers (a thin shell of porcelain, cemented over the front part of the tooth), and crowns. As a bonus, veneers or crowns can change the shape, size, and alignment of individual teeth.

"Only your dentist can determine which whitening method is most suitable for you," explains Dr. Veisman. "If you have many fillings, crowns, or bridges, you are not a suitable candidate for bleaching because the bleach will not change the color of fillings or dental porcelains. For darkly stained teeth and teeth with large fillings, veneers or crowns are the most appropriate whitening method."

Professionally bleached teeth will stay white for one to five years, depending on your diet and oral-hygiene habits. Smoking and drinking coffee and/or tea and red wine will necessitate "touchups" every six to twelve months. Do-it-yourself kits are not recommended. According to Dr. Veisman, the safest and most reliable bleaching comes with dentist-supervised home bleaching: "The trays fabricated by dentists are custom-made. They maximize contact with tooth structure while minimizing contact with the delicate gums. Poor-fitting trays can cause chemical burns to the gingivae. Furthermore, only dentists can prescribe and dispense concentrated carbamide peroxide solutions (10% to 16%) that will significantly lighten stained teeth."

The "whitestrips" sold in drugstores contain only 4.5-per-cent perox-ide. Because they are applied by a tape-like structure that does not tightly adapt to the curves of the teeth, it takes several weeks of wear to lighten within a shade category (so they are not for folks who want to go from yellow to white). Whitening toothpastes have the least lightening power because of their low concentration of ingredients and the minimal contact time with the teeth.

Dental implants are the most modern and aesthetically pleasing way of replacing a lost tooth. A dental implant is a titanium post that is embedded in the jawbone; a porcelain artificial tooth is then attached to the implant. Before dental implants, people could replace missing teeth only with uncomfortable dentures or bridges. Dentures can alter the sense of taste and speech and are extremely uncomfortable. They can also be dislodged quite easily and lead to embarrassment, especially if sneezed out at a family gathering. Dental bridges can fill gaps between teeth by joining healthy teeth together. However, this also entails cutting down perfectly good teeth in order to fill gaps, a process that is irreversible.

"Dental implants are clearly the best solution," says Dr. Veisman. "They improve one's appearance, are easy to look after, and maintain the integrity and health of the surrounding teeth. Most importantly, they allow for greater comfort and function, so that people can continue to enjoy the pleasures of life to the fullest."

While new dental-health procedures can make us look and feel better, Dr. Veisman reminds us that the basics are still important. She says, "Brush your teeth at least twice a day with fluoridated paste. Use soft-bristled toothbrushes exclusively, as other brushes abrade the protective enamel on teeth and contribute to gum recession. Use a gentle, circular massaging motion where the teeth and gums meet. Brushing the top of the tongue for a few seconds or using a 'tongue-scraper' removes the majority of bacteria responsible for breath odor. Spend three to four minutes to brush thor-oughly. Keep a toothbrush at work, especially if you have any porcelain veneers or crowns that you do not want to stain. Daily flossing is recom-mended, preferably at bedtime. There is an art to flossing, and your dentist can show you how to correctly floss if you are unsure. If you wear partial dentures, they should be removed and cleaned at bedtime."

It is important that boomers visit their dentists twice a year. With increased gum recession, men and women in midlife are more likely to develop root cavities. Your dentist will also check for cavities at the edges of older fillings, crowns, and bridges.

While individual situations and fees for specialists and labs vary, here are some approximate costs for the dental procedures discussed here:

- bleaching (home trays): $350 to $400
- veneers: $600 per tooth
- crowns: $850 per tooth
- implant: $3,000 per tooth, including surgical placement and porcelain crown

## A Weighty Matter

Both men and women in our survey identified weight gain as the most common change in their appearance in the last ten years, and the most difficult change to deal with. For those who were uncomfortable with their weight, nearby one-third wanted to lose between five and fifteen pounds – a goal that is probably attainable but hard to maintain. Those who aimed to lose more than this, including the 16 per cent who wanted to lose more than forty pounds, have a very big project ahead of them, and should seek the advice and help of their family physicians and/or accredited dietitians.

More than 70 per cent of our survey respondents had tried to lose weight in the last five to ten years. Since only one-quarter of them were advised to lose weight for medical reasons, it would seem that the majority wanted to lose weight for personal and aesthetic reasons. Unfortunately, when the motivation to lose weight is based largely on appearance, people often set unattainable goals that doom them to failure. "People need to understand that there is a healthy weight range based on your body-mass index that spans fifteen pounds or so," says Dr. Lhotsky. "I see so many people who want to lose thirty-five pounds and be right back to the low end of that range that they were at age twenty-five. In midlife, getting back into the upper end of the range – and losing fifteen pounds – may be a far more reasonable goal."

The national statistics show that boomer men are far more likely than boomer women to be overweight – and to suffer from diabetes and hypertension as a result. Ironically, although many men are concerned about this, women are far more likely than men to be taking steps to lose weight. "Let's face it," said one woman. "We learn early that thin girls are popular and fat girls are not; that happiness and love depend on how you look in a bathing suit. Even though we know this is an adolescent notion, it is a hard one to shake."

### SOME HIGHLIGHTS FROM THE HEALTHY BOOMER MIDLIFE SURVEY

---

*Are you comfortable with your current weight?*

| | |
|---|---|
| Yes | 35% |
| No | 65% |

---

*If you have tried to lose weight in the last year, what methods did you use?*

| | |
|---|---|
| Reduced calorie intake | 22% |
| Exercise | 21% |
| Reduced calorie intake and exercise combined | 49% |
| Weight loss program (e.g., Weight Watchers) | 10% |
| Diet drinks | 3% |
| Diet pills | 3% |
| Other | 5% |

---

Most of our survey respondents had made several attempts to lose weight. Some were unsuccessful. "I used to be able to lose five pounds easily when I was younger," said one woman, "but now those pounds just won't budge." After trying and failing many times, she gave up. "Maybe if I had a disease or needed an operation, then I would focus on losing weight." Others said they lost the weight, only to watch it creep back on at a disappointingly fast pace. As discussed in Chapter 2, maintaining change seems to be particularly difficult when it comes to managing weight. Many people who relapsed said that it was just too hard to discipline themselves in the face of daily temptations like delicious-looking desserts and time constraints that made them drop their regular exercise. One man admitted that he overate whenever he stopped writing down what went into his mouth. "As long as I use the Weight Watchers technique of honestly writing down everything I eat and stay aware of my point range on a weekly basis, I am fine. The minute I stop doing this, I am not aware of all the extras I am consuming. Within a week or two it starts to show on the scales." Repeated failures eventually wreak havoc on your self-efficacy (your belief that you can succeed). One woman said, "I have so much history with loss and gain that I figure the yo-yo syndrome is probably worse. So I have given up."

## Losing Weight: Dealing with the Barriers to Success

Why are losing weight and maintaining that loss so difficult for many people in midlife? One problem is unrealistic goal-setting, as discussed earlier. Studies repeatedly show that the initial goal should be to reduce the body weight by 10 per cent at a rate of one-half to one pound per week over the course of six months. That way you have a much better chance of maintaining the weight loss. While most of our respondents used a combination of a reduced-calorie-intake diet and exercise to lose weight, some talked about the futility of "lose weight quick" and fad-diet approaches. "I lost thirty pounds on the Atkins Diet," said one man, "but as soon as I went back to regular eating, I regained it all. I didn't have a plan for healthy eating and regular enjoyable physical activity that I could sustain over time." A woman told us how she crash-dieted and "cleansed" to look slim and trim at her daughter's wedding. Within two months she had regained all the weight.

Interestingly, many of the obstacles to success that our respondents identified may be rooted in physical and emotional problems that can be treated by your family doctor and psychotherapy. These include:

### Depression, Anxiety, and Burnout

Many people said that between job worries, financial concerns, and family pressures, they had no time or energy left to do the things they needed to do to lose weight. Dr. Lance Levy, a well-known specialist in eating disorders, has found that people who say they are desperate to lose weight but face these kinds of barriers are often suffering from undiagnosed anxiety, burnout, or depression. These conditions make it almost impossible for someone to lose weight and sometimes lead to binge-eating as a way to deal with loneliness, sadness, and other negative moods. When these conditions are relieved through the use of antidepressants and counseling, people are more likely to be able to move through the stages of change that will, in the end, lead to successful weight loss.

## Chronic Tiredness

One man said, "I know I would lose weight if I did not have to work so hard." Another woman talked about how she snacked and grazed in an effort to stay alert so she could work late and meet her deadlines. "It's become a habit to eat and drink almost continuously from 6:00 p.m. until I go to bed." Others talked about how feeling chronically tired meant that they moved around less in the day, and could not bring themselves to exercise. Ironically, those who did lose weight said that the biggest payoff and reinforcement to stay at a lower weight was "having more energy." One man said, "I used to feel drained at the end of the day and to puff when I climbed stairs. Now that I am fifteen pounds lighter and walking every day, I have a lot more energy." Midlife women and men who are chronically tired need to take a serious look at how well they are sleeping (see Chapter 1) and talk with their physicians about sleeping problems. Chronic tiredness leads to a vicious circle that disrupts our best efforts to reach and maintain a healthy weight.

## Chronic Pain

"I suffer a lot of fatigue and pain from fibromyalgia," said one woman, "so the last thing I want to do is exercise. I also use food to fend off the pain. Chocolate-chip cookies are my comfort food." If you suffer from chronic pain, ask your family physician for help with proper pain control so that you can begin to take action on losing weight.

## An Inability to Feel True Hunger

One man said, "An hour or two after a meal, I feel as if I have not eaten. Mentally, I know I have, but the hunger pangs are real to me." Dr. Levy and his colleagues have found that some people have difficulty differentiating between hunger and fullness because of gastrointestinal upsets such as reflux disease or queasy stomach. In an article in the *Canadian Journal of Diagnosis* in April 2000, he and his colleagues suggest that these symptoms prevent people from accurately listening to internal cues regarding hunger and thirst. Since learning to recognize hunger is essential to long-term weight control, people who suffer from heartburn, bloating, early satiety, constipation, diarrhea, and other symptoms of gastrointestinal upsets should talk with their family physicians about them.

In spite of all the barriers to weight management, some of our respondents succeeded in losing weight and maintaining the loss. When we asked them what worked, a couple of common themes surfaced. These included:

- Realistic weight-loss goals and a belief that they could be achieved
- A sustainable, long-term regimen that included healthy eating – not fad dieting – and moderate, regular exercise
- Support from family members and friends
- Small, consistent changes, such as eating sandwiches without butter or walking partway home from work every day
- Accountability systems, such as weighing in each week at Weight Watchers or a monthly weigh-in at your physician's office after the two of you have agreed on a weight-loss plan

## From the Research
### The Changing Face of Cosmetic Surgery

According to the American Society of Plastic Surgeons, between 1992 and 2000 the number of cosmetic-surgery procedures performed rose a dramatic 198 per cent. Since 1992, there has been a nearly 50 per cent increase in cosmetic-surgery procedures among men. In 2000, 14 per cent of all cosmetic-surgery procedures were performed on men.

Overall, the three most frequently requested of these are liposuction, breast augmentation, and improvement of the eyelids (blepharoplasty). Among men, nose reshaping (rhinoplasty) is the third most popular procedure.

Liposuction – the most popular procedure overall – is constantly being improved. For example, ultrasound-assisted liposuction is a relatively new form of liposuction that uses ultrasonography to target and remove fatty tissues more selectively and with minimal impact on surrounding tissues and blood vessels. Ultrasonic energy is used to fractionate, or burst, the fat cells. The fat is then removed with relatively low-volume suction, resulting in fewer traumas to tissues. Incisions, however, are larger.

There is also a trend towards women and men's opting for these surgical procedures at younger and younger ages. Instead of waiting until the signs of aging have become pronounced, many people now seek surgery in their late thirties or early forties to maintain their youthful appearance. This approach yields a subtle improvement rather than a dramatic change.

Source: American Society of Plastic Surgeons. *National Clearinghouse of Plastic Surgery Statistics* (2000). http://surgery.org

## Bionic Boomers

In the second half of the 1990s, the number of total knee- and hip-replacement operations performed in Canada soared. According to a report from the Canadian Institute for Health Information, this trend will likely continue as the large baby-boom generation ages.

There was a 45-per-cent increase in knee-replacement surgeries and a 19-per-cent increase in total-hip-replacement surgeries from 1994/95 to 1999/2000, the report revealed. The bulk of the operations – nearly 90 per cent – were performed on people aged fifty-five and older. The average hospital stay for these surgeries in 1999/2000 was ten days for a hip replacement and 8.5 days for a knee replacement.

Source: Canadian Institute for Health Information. *Canadian Joint Replacement Registry* (2002).

## On the Lighter Side

### Is That You?

A middle-aged woman had a heart attack and was taken to the hospital. While on the operating table, she had a near-death experience. Seeing God, she asked, "Is my time up?"

God said, "No, you have another forty years, two months, and eight days to live."

Upon recovery, the woman decided to stay in the hospital and have a facelift, liposuction, and a tummy tuck. Since she had so much more time left to live, she figured she might as well look her best.

After her last operation, she was released from hospital. While crossing the street on her way home, she was killed by an ambulance.

Standing before God, she demanded, "I thought you said I had another forty years? How come you didn't pull me out of the path of that ambulance?"

God replied, "Sorry. I didn't recognize you."

### Questions to Reflect On

Feelings about our physical appearance are complex and influenced by many factors, including cultural pressure, the degree of our self-esteem, and the response we get from partners, family members, and friends. Attractiveness and beauty are more about how we feel inside than what we see in the mirror.

1. What is one thing you can do to be more accepting of your physical appearance and more in tune with the internal gains you have made as you have grown older?
2. How do you plan to celebrate your next birthday as a positive marker in your journey through midlife?
3. Are you considering having a cosmetic procedure done (surgical or nonsurgical)? If yes, what do you expect to get out of it?
4. Are you trying to lose weight? If yes, do you have a reasonable weight-loss goal and a plan of action that make you feel that you will succeed? How ready are you to lose weight (see Chapter 2 to help you determine which Stage of Change you are in) and what one small, consistent step can you take now to move forward?

# CHAPTER SIX

# In the Kingdom of the Sick: Coping with Imperfect Health

Illness is the night-side of life, a more onerous citizenship. Everyone who is born holds dual citizenship, in the kingdom of the well and in the kingdom of the sick. Although we all prefer to use only the good passport, sooner or later each of us is obliged, at least for a spell, to identify ourselves as citizens of that other place.

— Susan Sontag, *Illness as Metaphor*, 1978

As we grow older, many boomers will become citizens of the kingdom of the sick, described by Susan Sontag above. Some of us will spend short periods of time there; others will spend years. Most of us arrive totally unprepared to live with the reality of imperfect health.

## An Ounce of Prevention

There are a lot of good reasons why our generation must do its best to prevent chronic illness. Obviously, the most important reason is personal. All of us want to remain healthy, independent, and involved in life. We also need to safeguard our universal health care system for future generations by keeping a lid on costs.

In the early decades of the twenty-first century the baby boomers – the largest cohort in Canadian history – will enter their senior years. If we experience the same incidence of diseases that previous generations have, our health-care system may not be able to meet the demand. Indeed, if there is no change in the per capita health-care expenditure and if the population ages as projected, the total per capita expenditure in Canada would be 31 per cent higher in 2030 than it is now, according to the *Health Policy Research Bulletin* (Vol. 1, Issue 1, March 2001).

Fortunately, experts predict that this will not happen. The boomers are healthier than previous generations, and disability and illness will likely be delayed or "compressed" into the last few years of their lives. (See "From the Research.")

Armed with this information and a pervasive belief that "it will never happen to me," most boomers are preoccupied with stopping the aging process, cheating time, and eliminating bulges in their bodies. But life is not always fair. Despite regular workouts and healthy eating, chronic illness can and does unexpectedly manifest itself. It is a rude awakening when someone who has pursued an active, healthy lifestyle is suddenly confronted with the limitations of illness and chronic disability.

One fifty-six-year-old woman described it this way. "I have always thought of myself as the 'queen of prevention.' My family would laugh at dinner – joking that, if they ate one more vegetable, they would turn into rabbits! Over the years, they learned to adapt and accept my persistence. They would not be surprised to find tofu in their birthday cakes. Exercise was part of my daily routine to deal with stress at work. My confidence in my invincibility reached its maximum when I declined the critical-care insurance offered to me a few weeks before I became ill. I told the agent, 'I do not need that insurance. I have good genes. I do everything right.'

"One week later I was diagnosed with malignant melanoma. Then, during the investigation to rule out the spread of the skin cancer, it was discovered that I had been exposed to tuberculosis. I was shocked. I could not believe that this was really happening to me. Sitting in the examination room, I felt the doctor must have been talking about somebody else, that this must be a bad dream. Then I had to wake myself up!

"My journey of illness was not to stop there. One month into taking medications for suspected tuberculosis, I developed severe side-effects. I was tired beyond what I ever knew tiredness could feel like. Now, I have liver damage, due to the drugs I was given for tuberculosis. I feel as if I have a huge balloon under my rib cage, when before I never even knew where my liver was.

"My perfect healthy life has changed. This has caused me to look at life differently. My priorities have shifted, and I now make an effort to live every day in the fullest possible way. Instead of worrying, I begin each morning thinking about what can be good about this day."

### Reality Check: Illness and Growing Older

**Mary** is a sixty-three-year-old woman who was well and very active until six months ago when she started to notice cramping and some weakness in her legs. One month later she developed pneumonia and, while hospitalized, was diagnosed with ALS, commonly called Lou Gehrig's disease. The next follow-up investigation showed that her pulmonary (lung) function had dropped dramatically, and that her vital capacity was now at 57 per cent of normal. In his report, the specialist said that Mary was at high risk for dying of respiratory failure during the night. Her prognosis was grave: 50 per cent of people die within three years of the onset of ALS.

Mary's story is just one example of what Dr. Lhotsky sees on a regular basis in the midlife health clinic. More and more, we are faced with the reality that aging and disease can often go hand in hand. Sometimes disease sneaks up slowly. But often, as in Mary's case, a quick and dramatic diagnosis seems to come out of nowhere. Here are some other examples:

- A fifty-four-year-old businesswoman, who has been constipated for three weeks, comes in with pain and a distended abdomen. She is admitted to hospital with a bowel obstruction that is later diagnosed as colon cancer. For now, she lives with a temporary colostomy, which will be reversed eventually, and faces chemotherapy for the cancer. While her prognosis for recovery is good, her quality of life has been dramatically altered.
- A forty-three-year-old teacher comes in complaining of unusual headaches that are different from her typical migraines. She is diagnosed with multiple sclerosis.
- A fifty-six-year-old businessman complains of a sudden onset of swollen ankles. He is diagnosed with chronic kidney disease and faces a possible need for kidney dialysis in the future.

All of these men and women will have to make significant changes in their lives in order to adapt and cope with a chronic illness.

## SOME HIGHLIGHTS FROM THE HEALTHY
## BOOMER MIDLIFE SURVEY

*Have you ever been diagnosed with a serious long-term condition (e.g., diabetes, arthritis, cancer)?*

| | |
|---|---|
| No | 67% |
| Yes | 31% |
| No answer | 2% |

*Are you taking any long-term medications?*

| | |
|---|---|
| No | 55% |
| Yes | 41% |
| No answer | 4% |

Slightly fewer than one-third of the respondents to the Healthy Boomer Midlife Survey said they had been diagnosed with a serious long-term illness. This is similar to the findings of Canada's large 1996/97 National Population Health Survey. It also shows significant differences between men and women. Women aged forty-five to sixty-five are more likely than men to be dealing with arthritis (26%), hypertension (18%), and migraines (12%). Midlife men, on the other hand, are more likely to be coping with heart disease (6%) and diabetes (6%).

Some have reached a stage of acceptance of their diseases and have taken steps to adapt, like this fifty-year-old man: "I have arthritis in my hips. I have gone from running to biking and continue strength training. I will miss my daily runs, but feel the biking will serve effectively in its place. I am learning to accept and appreciate all the other positive changes in my life." After developing arthritis in her feet, a fifty-five-year-old woman told us she had to give up tap-dancing, a childhood passion she had picked up again in her late forties. However, she stays active with power-walking, squash, and working out with weights.

Forty-one per cent of our survey's respondents were taking prescription medication. The most common were hormone therapy and medications to treat thyroid problems, depression, and hypertension, and to help control pain associated with fibromyalgia and arthritis. Many boomers are unhappy about this. Ironically, the generation that was quick to try recreational drugs hates to take prescription ones. "I can't stand being on pills" and "I want to get drug-free" are refrains we hear often in our clinic. The Big Generation hates to be reminded by a daily pill that we do not always reside in the kingdom of the well.

### Accepting, Adapting, and Coping

When **Joyce** developed breast cancer, her previous concerns about wrinkles suddenly seemed frivolous. Now she was dealing with the outcomes of surgery, fatigue, depressed moods, and fear of death. She knew she had to go on living and adapt to her new situation. Dealing with the physical problems was hard enough. "I had to change my self-image," she said. "I wasn't my energetic self any more, and I had no new me to replace the old. I worried that I would be a burden to my partner and he would find me unattractive, that I'd be socially isolated."

Slowly but surely, she accepted the loss of her old self. She forged a new one with different expectations of what she could accomplish in a day. She stopped going to "empty" cocktail parties and concentrated on being with friends and family members that she cared about. She learned to find joy in small things.

Boomers who are fortunate enough to live in the kingdom of the well know they can learn a lot from Joyce and others who live with chronic illness. But too often the response to Joyce's story is "Good for her . . . but it won't happen to me. I'll stop and smell the roses next year, after I get over this major piece of work . . . or after my son graduates . . . or after I pay off the mortgage."

Illness does not always wait for a graduation to be over or a mortgage to be paid. Sometimes there are few or no warning signs; sometimes, mild symptoms sneak up on you. Often, the diagnosis is a shock, as it was for Fran.

**Fran** describes her experience with chronic illness in midlife. "The winter I turned fifty I noticed I was having difficulty making my turns while I was downhill skiing with my family. Within a few months I was sitting in a neurologist's office with my husband. I heard the shattering first few sentences: 'Do you live in a two-story house or a bungalow? You will be disabled in five years. You have Parkinson's disease.'

"We walked out numb, feeling shocked. My husband hugged me and told me that, no matter what happened, he would always be there for me. We needed to get some information about Parkinson's disease (PD) right away. We walked directly across the street to the Parkinson Society. They were very kind and calming, and gave me a book to read about the disease.

"After a few months, I saw a PD specialist and quickly started to feel better. I agreed to participate in a new drug trial. I felt supported by the staff. I felt they cared how I was feeling and I got a lot more positive information.

"I was not going to let this illness stop me from living. I was half finished my Ph.D. program. I knew I had to keep going and be strong. I have two teenage children. I did not want them to feel they had an invalid, grandmother-like mom! I had a great inspiration in my own mother, who fought cancer with four surgeries. She was very strong, and I determined that I would be, too.

"We still do everything together as a family, but I have to adjust my activities. So now I do not downhill-ski. When the family hits the slopes, I go cross-country skiing. Often, my son and husband come with me for part of the day.

"The hardest part of living with a chronic illness is the *losses*. I had to give up driving; I did not feel safe. I am presently participating in a fitness program, and I realize that I am not improving like all the others in the program, I am just maintaining! This can be frustrating at times, because I work very hard.

"I read about my disease on a need-to-know basis only. I went to one conference about PD, but I found it scary to see people at the various stages of the disease. I try to always find some humor to help me deal with stressful situations like these. They served us linguini at lunch, with a very small fork. Suddenly all the participants at my table started to laugh, when we saw each other struggling to eat linguini with our shaking hands.

"I find some of the websites about PD overwhelming, although I know the chat groups may help some people. I have my own support group, not related to my illness. The members of the group are always understanding; I can share my worries and frustrations.

"Although I am officially retired, I still work almost full-time. But I do it at my pace. I take the mornings off for my fitness. I have my own consulting business and I teach a graduate program at the University of Ottawa. I always try to deal with my 'clumsiness' with a bit of humor. I tell the students that I have Parkinson's disease, so they are not worried that my tremor is due to nervousness.

"I know I have a progressive illness, but you can adapt your life to deal with this. I think of other people who have more serious conditions. Mine is manageable; I just have to be careful. I keep telling myself, 'Be easy on yourself.' Looking ahead is not a productive thing for me to do. I do not know when things will deteriorate, so I am living each day as it comes. Attitude is important. You have to stay planted in the present."

The research confirms what Fran knows. Courage, living in the present, making small adjustments in daily life, and staying close to family and friends are effective coping strategies when illness strikes.

Concentrating on today and mutual support between loving partners is a key feature of how **Joanne** and her husband **Tom** adapt and cope with chronic illness. Joanne is a fifty-six-year-old architect. She was diagnosed with cardiomyopathy at age twenty-seven, only three years after she graduated from university, and she was fitted with a pacemaker. Her heart condition did not stop her from pursuing an active life for the next twenty years. She went to Abu Dhabi a few years later to work, where she met and fell in love with her future husband. They traveled back to Canada together via a trip around the world and settled in Toronto.

Joanne says, "Everything changed in 1993 when I suffered a stroke at age forty-seven. I had trouble speaking and writing and had weakness on my right side. I was in rehabilitation for many months. When I started back to work, it was difficult to cope, though I tried very hard to pretend that all was normal. Eventually the project I was working on got canceled and I lost my job.

"For two years I tried to get a new job. I sent over a hundred letters and called everyone on my contact list, but I still had the speech problem. I decided to get a degree in commerce but, when I was halfway through, I realized how much the stroke had affected me. I had to admit I could not do it.

"My next project was to open my own business in conference planning. I took a course in conference planning and got ready. But I could not get it going. My fantasies that everyone would 'overlook' my stilted speech were wrong. I took a different course, this time in desktop publishing, and finally landed a job. But within four months, I was in a hospital again! My cardiomyopathy had progressed into congestive heart failure, and to top it off I was diagnosed with myasthenia gravis. I am now on a list for a heart transplant and waiting for my condition to deteriorate. This could take three weeks, three months, three years, or even thirty years.

"I had to accept that things were changing. I could not go camping, skiing, or hiking or do my usual activities. I increased my reading substantially. Walking a few blocks was now a major effort.

"But I am not giving up. I just started cardiac rehab. I feel that maybe it is possible to strengthen my own body and be able to 'bounce back' from the surgery. I am sure that it is better to have your own heart if you can. Sometimes all of this gets me down and I feel sad. I have had so many losses. But on my better days, I realize I still have a good life.

"Since my 'healthy' husband suffered an angina attack recently, paradoxically, our illnesses have brought a special closeness to our marital relationship.

"This summer we went to our weekend place up north. We bought a small boat with a motor so we could go out on the lake. We fished, read on the boat, slipped in for a quick swim – we had so much fun together. My husband is now fixing up the weekend place and working on an addition. I still go for my walks in the woods, but now I take my cell phone with me, just in case.

"I do not think about the future, because I know my heart will deteriorate. I think of *now*, maybe one week ahead. So when Christmas is coming, I do not think about my illness, but of the celebration and how best to enjoy it.

"My husband took early retirement and we've sold our three-level home for a condo on the lakefront with plenty of parks and activities around. We're getting a dog and will spend more time at our weekend place. Life is different, of course, but it is not the end! The key is to find something that interests both of you that you can act on now, knowing that you will get sick at some point that's *not* convenient to you! But this is what a supportive family is for."

By coincidence, the terrorist attacks in New York and Washington happened three days before journalist and media personality **Pamela Wallin** underwent surgery for colon cancer. The tragedy of September 11, 2001, dramatically influenced her thoughts and attitude, both before and after the surgery.

Pamela says, "Going to New York made me realize I was being given a second chance; those poor people in the towers had no chance. I came back emotionally changed. I began to let go of things that are not important – all the stress, all the battles and frustrations – the 'poison' that had manifested itself through the cancer. It was time to let it go. It was invigorating to realize that life is about deciding what matters the most. This was an important part of the healing process for me."

Initially, it was difficult for Pamela, who is driven by her work and boundless curiosity, to accept the diagnosis. "I think it was a combination of shock and fear. I have a mind trained to manage crisis and unexpected situations – it comes with my job. So I reacted as if it were a news story. Get the facts. And I had immediate questions. How am I going to tell my parents? How will I manage my career with cancer in my life? I need to work; I have shows to do. This is my livelihood. There were many questions about death as well, but only in the middle of the night. I am an insomniac, so that is often when big issues like that would come to mind . . ."

Waiting for surgery was not easy. "When you are diagnosed with cancer you become obsessed with getting it out of your body. I was told there were two people ahead of me. They were younger and, therefore, their conditions more urgent. Waiting lists are a big issue when it comes to cancer. You begin to understand quickly about the problems in our system, like the staffing shortages in hospitals. It was comforting – and necessary – to have my family around. My father, who is a former X-ray technician, understood the hospital system, and he intervened on a couple of crucial occasions."

After she recovered from surgery, she immediately embarked on a book tour. She made few modifications to her hectic schedule. "I did not change anything drastically, just small things such as scheduling a day off between flights to different time zones and having more quiet time. My sister came with me to help. As a public person, people are always calling me: could you speak here, address this conference, and so on. I am learning I can – sometimes – say no to the external world."

Pamela quit smoking before the surgery. Now she is "trying to be sensible, to eat better, take better care of myself, and learn to prioritize." She also decided to speak publicly about her experience with colon cancer. This is a great service to the rest of us, most of whom do not want to discuss cancer at all, let alone this particular type. "I had to admit my own ignorance about colon cancer. I did not know how common it was, that it affected women, not just men."

Her openness has been rewarded. "Since I have spoken out, I have received a lot of letters, some saying they were praying for me, others sharing their experiences, others offering encouragement. This has been wonderful, particularly when people tell me they are motivated to go for a test."

What advice does Pamela give to other boomers who are diagnosed with a serious illness? "Be in tune with your body, pay attention to changes or symptoms and go have them checked. We are so busy in our lives, we often forget to listen to our bodies."

She also practices what research has confirmed: people who stay in control and refuse to see themselves as victims cope better and stay healthier. "Gone are the days of being told what to do," Pamela says. "You have to be your own advocate. I had to do my own research and call people I knew to help me make decisions. I am fortunate, because years of investigative journalism have made me familiar with how to do this. Stay in charge; you have to know what is going on at all times, so that you can make conscious choices."

**From the Research**
*Living Longer with Fewer Disabilities (Compressed Morbidity)*
Most of us remember how our grandparents accepted the fact that they would live with disabilities, such as hearing loss and arthritis, in their sixties and early seventies. Today, many boomers can postpone these disabilities until the final years of their lives.

Dr. James Fries, a world expert on aging and disability, has shown that, over the last thirty years, the length of time older adults in North America can expect to live without disabilities has increased significantly. In other words, the onset of disabilities associated with aging and illness has been "compressed" to the later years of life.

There are likely a number of reasons for this, including higher incomes and better medical interventions, as well as positive changes in the way we live. Fries and his colleagues have followed 1,741 Stanford University alumni for almost forty years. The subjects were put into high-, moderate-, and low-risk categories based on smoking, weight, and exercise patterns. People in the high-risk category in 1962 and 1986 had twice the level of disability in 1998 that those in the low-risk category had. His conclusion: not only do people with better health habits live longer, but also disability is potentially compressed into the later years of life.

Source: Vita, A., R. B. Terry, H. B. Hubert, and J. F. Fries. "Aging, Health Risks and Cumulative Disability." *New England Journal of Medicine* (1998).

*Changing Patterns in Chronic Disease*

The prevalence of many chronic conditions among Canadians in midlife (ages forty-five to sixty-four) has declined over the last twenty years. As a result, people aged sixty-five to seventy-four are less likely to be limited in their activities than were their parents' or grandparents' generations. But the prevalence of some conditions has increased in midlife. Asthma has increased among both men and women; diabetes has increased significantly in men, and midlife women are more likely to have migraines. The greater number of diabetic men in midlife is likely linked to weight gain and sedentary living, as well as improved methods of detecting the disease.

Source: Statistics Canada. "How Healthy Are Canadians?" *Health Reports*, Vol. 11, No. 3 (Winter 1999).

**Questions to Reflect On**

As we have seen in this chapter, there are no guarantees. Practicing a healthy lifestyle in midlife will not necessarily increase how long we will live – quantity – but it will likely improve the quality of the years you have ahead, whether or not you are living with a chronic illness or disability. Boomers who are fortunate enough to live in the kingdom of the well can learn a lot from the courage and philosophy of peers who are living with chronic illness. We can all benefit from applying their strategies for accepting, adapting, and coping.

1. What would you do differently if you were diagnosed with a chronic or life-threatening disease?
2. What's stopping you from doing this now?
3. What is one step you could take to make this change now?

# CHAPTER SEVEN

# Will My Money Run Out Before I Do?

If I were a rich man
I'd have the time that I lack
To sit in the Synagogue and pray . . .
That would be the sweetest thing of all.
> – Jerry Bock, Sheldon Harnick, *Fiddler on the Roof*, 1964

Like the main character in *Fiddler on the Roof*, most boomers believe that, if they were rich, they would have the time they now lack to pursue their dreams and rediscover their true selves. But the anxiety and the long hours we work to pursue financial dreams are the very traps that get in the way of our doing what we most want and need to do at this time in our lives. "I am at the height of my earning power," explained one man. "Now is the time I need to work my buns off to make enough for my kids' education, my mother's nursing home, and my own retirement. The problem is that when I work this hard, I don't have time to enjoy life, especially time with my family. I feel anxious a lot of the time. I don't want to live this way, but I feel like I have no choice."

This chapter is about what money, work, and retirement mean to us, and how they are linked with the almost universal feeling boomers express of being constantly "time-crunched."

### Financial Fears

At this stage of life, making money is as important for women as it is for men. Most believe that they will outlive their partners and the "bag lady" fear nags at them. "It might sound irrational," said one fifty-three-year-old woman, "but I live in fear of being old and alone, living in an upstairs flat, eating cat food." The woman who said this has a good job but a very small pension because she took time off to raise her children. Her husband is self-employed and lost most of his retirement investment when his business went under five years ago. "I can't count on my husband to look after me," she says, "and I have a lot of catching up to do on RRSPs. Retirement is just not in the cards for me for a very long time."

Fifty-year-old **Jennifer** feels particularly vulnerable, because she has no children. She explains, "I don't have any kids to help me when I am old. I need to earn enough now so that I can look after myself later." Paradoxically, she and other boomers we talked with worry about financial security even though they are economically privileged beyond the wildest dreams of their Depression-era parents. This can make it difficult to be realistic about planning for an uncertain future. Jennifer happily donates 10 per cent of what she earns to her church and international charity work. "I know I am privileged," she asserts. "Financially, I have so much more than my own mother had. Giving with joy allows me to receive with joy. I never resent this."

**Joanne Thomas Yaccato** is the bestselling author of *Balancing Act: A Canadian Woman's Financial Success Guide* (1994) and *Raising Your Business: A Canadian Woman's Guide to Entrepreneurship* (1998). She is also the president and founder of Women and Money Inc. We talked with her about women's fears of outliving their money. She had this to say: "We have to keep reminding ourselves that one out of three women retiring at sixty-five will be living at the poverty line or lower. The 1950s idea of marrying your financial plan has not worked out for most women. While it's changing for younger women, I still meet twenty-year-olds who have the same bag-lady fears as midlife women. They see their mothers and grandmothers struggling to make ends meet. Fear is the great inhibitor, more than a lack of education or bad financial planning. It's what interferes with us being financially successful."

Some women are taking chances in new careers and self-employment in midlife. We asked Joanne what the important issues are here:

"Like everything else in life, we think about things differently than men do. Women have become much greater risk-takers. Women are opening businesses three times as often as men in Canada. Many have run into the glass ceiling in corporate Canada. It's very important for women to ask themselves, 'What is this business for?' Be clear about what you want and need in terms of emotional as well as financial returns."

When we asked her what advice she would give to boomer women, she replied: "There is a lot of good news. Never before has there been so much pertinent information for women about finance. Just make sure that, if you're looking for a book on finances, you buy one specifically for women. There are two great motivators for women to get savvy about money. The first is divorce or the death of a spouse; the second is finally having the time to study. Don't wait that long! As women, we are not socialized to be competent about money. I often joke with women that, financially, we need to become the men we wished we had married! I think one of the greatest gifts I can give my daughter is financial literacy."

The 2001 Healthy Boomer Midlife Survey confirmed the findings of our initial study in 1999. Financial security, followed closely by illness, was the most common worry about life after retirement. Fewer than one-third of the respondents said that they felt financially ready for retirement, even though most did prepare for retirement by purchasing Registered Retirement Savings Plans. The same findings were confirmed in the large MacArthur Foundation Research Study of 1999 that examined some eight thousand Americans in midlife. In this study, the two areas over which people in midlife felt they had the least control were finances and sexual activity.

In their efforts to gain control and financial security in old age, many boomers have invested heavily in the market, especially in mutual funds and stocks. Wild rides in high-tech stocks, economic crises in Asia and South America, and a series of recessions in North America have eroded our sense of financial security and hence our sureness about our own futures. Downturns resulting from unpredictable events, especially the terrorist acts of September 11, 2001, have further heightened this sense of insecurity. For some, the financial fallout of September 11 has been devastating. For many, the tragedy has led them to reflect on what is really important in life. "I guess my life is as good as it is going to get in terms of work, money, health, and family," said one man. "I hope I can learn to enjoy and embrace it more fully – before it begins changing for the not-so-good or worse."

SOME HIGHLIGHTS FROM THE HEALTHY
BOOMER MIDLIFE SURVEY

| *Do you feel financially secure?* | |
| --- | --- |
| Yes | 48% |
| No | 46% |
| Do not know | 6% |

| *Do you plan to retire?* | |
| --- | --- |
| Gradually | 49% |
| All at once | 20% |
| Not at all | 21% |

| *Do you feel financially prepared for retirement?* | |
| --- | --- |
| Yes | 32% |
| No | 55% |
| Do not know | 12% |

## Working Longer, Working Harder

Making money in the prime of our lives is a key motivator for working longer and harder. "The lifestyle we have is expensive," said one fifty-two-year-old man, "so backing off on the workload is not an option at this time. I work long hours. The buck stops at my desk. If I mess up, the firm and the employees are at risk. I try to delegate and find time to mentor the bright stars, but until I can satisfy the flow of money we need now and in the future I have no choice but to work long and hard."

Remember the prediction in the 1960s that technology was going to give us more hours of recreation and less of work? Somewhere along the way, this failed to happen. In fact, the reverse has come to pass. North Americans still work about the same number of hours as their parents did and, for some midlife men and women, those hours have increased, sometimes dramatically. "I always have too much work to complete," said one woman, "although I know my perfectionism is part of the problem."

Work and family-life conflicts are related to overload, unrealistic expectations, and pressures to meet deadlines. "Work will always fill the time available," said one man. "You have to realize that you can only do so much." Another woman spoke of the need to set priorities. She said, "Deal with one issue at a time and don't feel guilty that you are only human." Another man said, "I try to address problems immediately rather than let them build up. However, I need to learn how to take breaks during the day and incorporate relaxation techniques into my life."

A recent study by the Canadian Policy Research Networks based on two large national surveys confirmed that increased workloads are the norm in the twenty-first century. The average employee in Canada spent forty-five hours a week in paid employment in 2001, compared to forty-two hours in 1991. High stress on the job was identified by survey respondents twice as often as ten years ago.

Studies show that, in all age groups, men tend to spend more hours than women do in paid employment. However, women spend more time than men in unpaid work such as childcare, meal preparation, and housework. When the two are added up, women typically spend more hours than men working. "My biggest challenge is to juggle my work and family life," said one woman in her mid-forties. "There are never enough hours to do what is demanded of me."

A recent Statistics Canada study showed that working long hours in paid work – an average of fifty-one to fifty-five hours per week – was more common among men aged twenty-five to forty-four than among men aged forty-five and older. This means that men with young children are the least likely to have enough time to spend with their families.

**Bill** is president of a financial-consulting company and the father of two children aged four and six. He works fifty-five to sixty hours a week or more.

"At my level, this is expected," he explains. "I have a good income but do not feel financially secure yet. To support the family and keep the lifestyle we enjoy, I have to work long hours. It's a vicious circle. When there is an economic downturn, my work gets slower and I have more time with my family, but I earn less money. It's all a function of how the economy per-forms. If the economy is going well, I could retire in five years.

"I am good at my work and I have a strong work ethic. But in my busi-ness, you are only as good as the last job you did. You have to guard your reputation. If I could afford it, I would take a lower position, but if I apply for a lower-paid job with shorter hours, a potential employer will ask, Why? What is wrong? There have been some opportunities for less-stressful jobs that have a good salary, but we would have to move.

"I don't get to see my children on weekday mornings, and I am seldom home for dinner. I try to compensate by taking them to soccer and swimming, skating and skiing on the weekends. I carry them to bed at night, just to have some precious time with them.

"My children are very important to me. I want them to have more than I did when I was young. I did not have a lot growing up. My first job was doing manual labor in a boiler room.

"I don't have much time left over for myself, but I don't need a lot either. I am kind of a solitary person. I relax by watching TV, chopping wood, and being at home. My wife and I enjoy going out for dinners and visiting friends. Sometimes in the summer, I like having a beer on the terrace at home . . ."

In contrast to men, the proportion of women who work long hours tends to increase with age – from 26 per cent in the twenty-five to thirty-four age group, to 30 per cent in the forty-five to fifty-four age group. Some midlife women may be working longer hours because their children have grown up and left home, others because they have advanced in their careers and are now eager to take on more responsibility at work. Still others, especially those who are single or childless, may need to work long hours to build financial security.

One woman said, "I have a lot of fun in both roles, but I find it hard to make the transition. When I am at work or in a work mindset, it is hard to switch to dealing with teenage concerns. I have a tendency to spend too many hours working, but I work hard to enjoy time at home. I rarely take work home. A great partner helps a lot, too!"

Boomers use some novel strategies to help make the transition from work to home. Forty-five-year-old Carol, who is the mother of two small children, described the first thing she does when she comes in the front door from work. She gets down to eye level with her toddler and first-grader. They spend five minutes hugging and whispering together about how the day has gone. "Then they run off. I gather up my purse and briefcase and take a big breath. I have made the transition." In this way, Carol eases the transition for herself and her children to have a calmer, easier evening together.

A man who worked from his home office explained on CBC Radio how each morning he put on his coat, went out the back door, and came in the front door to begin working in his home office. He did the reverse in the evening. Until he started this routine, he said it was almost impossible to separate work and home life and to really "be there" for his wife and children at the end of the day.

### Rewards and Challenges

More than three-quarters of our respondents said they were "very" or "somewhat satisfied" with their work lives. Some told us that accomplishing things at work was one of their greatest joys in midlife. They spoke about feeling good because they now have the wisdom and experience they need to succeed and forge ahead in their careers.

Clearly, work is an important source of well-being and self-esteem for many people in midlife. We heard repeatedly that the challenge was to find a balance between time spent with family, work, and self.

For the boomers in our survey who were unhappy at work, job dissatisfaction centered on feeling undervalued and insufficiently supported by managers and bosses. One woman said, "I try to deal with this by keeping communication lines open with my manager." Others said they relied on supportive family members and friends to reinforce their self-worth. A few people talked about pressures to keep up with younger employees who have advanced technical skills.

To some extent, our respondents' concerns reflect bigger problems that will affect all ages. As the largest generation in history prepares to retire – or to not retire – they also feel a growing anger and frustration with what they see as age discrimination and the business world's failure to make changes that accommodate older workers and make the best use of their talents.

The doom-and-gloom prediction that our pension scheme will collapse and our children will slave to support the boomers when they retire en masse is largely based on scaremongering. Nonetheless, the North American economy needs to encourage older workers – typically defined as fifty-five-plus – to continue to work, not to chase them away with early-retirement plans and biased perceptions that older workers cannot adapt.

Many older workers want to work differently. "I want to continue to work," said one man, "but I am tired of the grind. I want to work less hours and have more time for family and personal growth." Others talked about the desire to mentor, pass on their knowledge, and upgrade their skills. The fifty-five-and-older crowd wants more-flexible work hours, increased opportunities for telecommuting, and computer screens that are easier on aging eyes.

A number of people talked about new careers they had embarked on in midlife or how they had switched to self-employment after leaving jobs they had been in for a long time. This appears to be a growing trend for our generation. Downsizing and early-retirement plans have enabled many boomers to recast themselves as consultants or to start their own businesses. However, some described themselves as discouraged and still looking. "I haven't been able to find permanent work because I am considered 'too senior' for many roles. As a former C.E.O., I am used to big-picture thinking, but companies are looking more for depth in one area."

"The sudden decline in the high-tech industry has hurt a lot of boomers," explained one human-resources consultant. "For the first time, companies are laying off senior people who are really valuable employees. In the past, these people were relatively immune to cutbacks."

While many senior people suffer depression and other stress-related conditions when they are laid off, **Alan** relies on a positive attitude and family support to bounce back.

He is a senior director of marketing in a large company where he continues to reinvent himself in new jobs, in response to corporate restructuring. Alan says, "In advertising, we say that, if you have not been fired at least twice, you are not working hard enough. I change jobs about every five years. I always have a game plan when I change jobs. I look for something that interests me and will help me learn new things."

His wife Frances plays an important role in how Alan deals with these changes. "You have to know what your priorities are," he says. "With Frances and me, family and our relationship come first. I remember working for Coca-Cola and they used to say, 'If the company wanted you to have a wife, they would have given you one!' But I say, 'I have a wife, I can always get a job!'

"It is a mistake not to tell your wife and family that you have lost a job and are looking for another one. When I call my long list of contacts, I have to be up on the phone. Frances keeps me in this positive frame of mind."

One person spoke about the challenges of self-employment. "Being self-employed can be isolating at times. I have to work at maintaining contacts to ensure that I have access to an outside sounding board and to advice and training. I stay connected via an online network and I keep in touch with my former employer. Sharing work and training costs with other consultants helps a lot."

### Losing a Business: Finding Another Way

In some cases, like that of **Valerie** and **Noel**, the economic recession of the early 1990s acted as their impetus to forge new careers while in their fifties. When they shut down their clothing-design and import business in 1994, retiring was not possible. They had two daughters in high school and no corporate pension plan. Both of them now agree that the change turned out to be the best thing that could have happened.

When they closed their business, **Valerie** decided to upgrade the skills she had used in her former career as a librarian. She signed up for an advanced nine-month program in computer technology.

"It was intensive and exhausting," she says. "I knew virtually nothing about computers. I hadn't taken math since Grade 12 and here I was learning to build systems and program in computer language. I knew I was over my head, but I also knew that I needed the qualifications to be credible. I was the oldest person in the class. Most of my classmates were in their late twenties and had been using computer technology most of their lives."

She admits that she was frightened. She questioned her abilities and had moments of despair. But quitting or failing was just not an idea she would entertain. "I worked from 4:30 a.m. to midnight. I cried a lot. Noel was always there to hold me and tell me that I could do it."

After graduation, she became a successful communications consultant working with a series of long-term contracts with high-tech companies. She forged an exciting new career by combining her information management and technology skills with her experience in business and her natural ability to get along with people. "I am very happy with how it turned out," says Valerie. "In a family business you are never sure what your contribution is. Now, I feel more in control and satisfied, knowing that I can make it on my own."

She believes that overcoming fears of inadequacy and negative self-esteem can be major hurdles for women in midlife. "Women should never underestimate the value of their business and life experience."

What is Valerie's advice to others who decide to change gears in midlife? "Don't be afraid to invest in yourself at any age. You have a lot of skills to offer that you are probably not even aware of. Be prepared to retrain and to be flexible in how you use your new skills. Go for what presents itself. It's a wonderful feeling to forge a new career."

Initially, **Noel** found it very difficult to leave the family business. "It was what I had done for twenty-three years. It was part of my identity and my security," he says. "At the same time, I had the feeling I was becoming fossilized. My brain was getting soggy. I wasn't learning much doing the same thing over and over. In an unexpected way, the economic recession was my salvation. The business just was not viable, so I was forced to change."

Noel had always had an interest in investing, and he had handled the money in the family business. For the next two years, he kept one foot in the clothing business, working for other companies, and the other foot in dedicating his time to learning more about investing. While he was taking the Canadian Securities course, his professor introduced him to Jack, an established investment advisor in a large company. Jack became his mentor and encouraged him to become an investment advisor with his firm.

"I believe the company had some reservations about hiring a fifty-two-year-old," says Noel, "because they need to invest in a new advisor for two years or more until you can build up a clientele. Yet Jack and I both knew that I would have more credibility with clients than younger people because of my years of experience in business and personal investing."

Noel is now well established in the company. "Best of all is the stimulation and learning opportunities I have found in this new career," he asserts. "I am learning every day, and the old sense of feeling stagnant is totally gone."

He helps manage the stress of his current job with a regular fitness routine and daily meditation sessions. His advice for other boomers considering a life change? "Take the challenge gladly. It is an opportunity to learn and grow. Go for it."

As individuals and as a couple, Valerie and Noel managed to convert the negative experience of losing a business into a positive growth experience. They readily admit that making these career changes took time, persistence, and effort. Starting new careers in midlife is not easy, but it is possible. Their stories show how important it is to recognize and have confidence in the experience and skills you have built up over the years.

### SOME HIGHLIGHTS FROM THE HEALTHY BOOMER MIDLIFE SURVEY

*How satisfied are you with your work life?*

| | |
|---|---|
| Very satisfied | 37% |
| Somewhat satisfied | 39% |
| Neither satisfied nor dissatisfied | 8% |
| Somewhat dissatisfied | 3% |
| Very dissatisfied | 5% |
| No answer | 8% |

*Do the stresses you experience related to work lead to unhealthy behaviors?*

| | |
|---|---|
| Yes | 45% |
| No | 44% |
| No answer | 11% |

## Searching for Balance

The vast majority of people we see at our clinic and those we interviewed said it was a major challenge to achieve balance in their personal, work, and family lives. One fifty-year-old woman said, "I'm certainly aware of the need for a more balanced life, but with a young child, a busy career, commuting, and elderly parents, it seems more a dream than a reality. I am always thinking I need some time away from it all to look at my priorities, but I never seem to be able to give that to myself." Inevitably, both women and men who combine long work hours and responsibilities at home feel squeezed, with no time for themselves. This was most apparent for those in the sandwich group, who have both child and eldercare responsibilities. The younger the child or children, the higher the incidence of role overload.

We asked boomers how they dealt with the challenge of overload and of striking a balance between work, family, and self-care. Joanne Thomas Yaccato said that, to ensure some quality of life, she contracts out a lot of things. As an entrepreneur, she took "a major financial hit" by hiring someone who functions as a general manager of her business and as a personal assistant. This gives her more time with her young daughter. "But," she adds, "I still don't feel balanced. I still do the lion's share of home and childcare. Maybe I'm just plain pissed off. I also know I need a spiritual connection. That would help me feel balanced, but mostly I'm just too tired."

We asked **Margot Franssen**, president and partner of The Body Shop Canada, how she achieves balance in her life among work, home, and self-care. She recently turned fifty and is the mother of three teenagers aged fourteen, fifteen, and seventeen.

Like many boomers we spoke with, Margot says, "My biggest problem has always been finding time for me. Everyone else's needs would come first. I had a bad back problem a few years ago that forced me to make more time for myself. This led me to realize that I could work more from home, and that has turned out to be a good thing for me and my family. E-mail is my savior."

Margot says she takes care of herself by setting certain guidelines. "I tend not to work nights or weekends," she says. "When I do go flat out for a week, I am generally on the road. When I'm home, I'm home for me."

The family takes holidays, like river-rafting, where "there's no possible way people can reach me." These experiences where she "knows nothing and doesn't have to pretend to know," and where she puts herself in the hands of the trip guides really "realign and rejuvenate" her. She also readily admits to the satisfying and instantly gratifying experience of computer games to take her mind away from work issues.

Suggestions from our survey respondents seemed to come down to two key messages:

- Reframe your priorities, and
- Make a clear commitment.

*Reframing Priorities*

We often shift the focus of our priorities because of a major life event or a sudden realization. Joanne made the step toward more balance by hiring a manager when her daughter was born. Another woman said, "I looked at what I really wanted out of life and I went for it. I didn't want a tombstone that said, 'Here lies a lonely woman who worked herself to death.'" Another man said, "I just got tired of working long hours to build the perfect picket fence for my children and decided to enjoy them now." A single parent told us that when she realized that she felt "like a gerbil running around on a wheel," she looked for small changes she could make so she could have some free time to be with adult friends.

For some, the motivation for change is an illness or conflict in the family. One man said that he had to develop more balance between work and home when his partner developed a chronic illness and required his support and strength, as well as his wages. Another man talked of facing the fact that he lived with a lot of family friction. Through a lengthy process of family meetings, he and his wife and kids reached an agreement to reduce stress by purchasing fewer things and devoting more time to simple activities with family and friends.

*Making a Commitment*

Committing to change and taking action are difficult tasks for most of us. They mean moving beyond just thinking about doing something, and many boomers just don't know how to do that. The Strategic Coach Program, developed by **Dan Sullivan** and his partner **Babs Smith**, helps entrepreneurs move beyond this place, and offers useful ideas for everyone.

This highly successful Program consists of a one-day seminar every three months for a minimum of three years. In this way, participants establish a habit of making regular times for reflection, reorganization, and goal-setting. It provides what most of us don't willingly commit to – time away from home and the office when we can plan ways to improve the quality of our own lives, as well as that of our families. The Program helps participants divide their time into days to work at what they do best and earn income, while they delegate everything else, days to clean up messes, learn new skills, etc., and days that are totally free of work. There is an emphasis on increasing the number of work-free days. Dan and Babs avidly practice what they teach, taking fourteen weeks a year for holidays.

Some of the tenets of the Strategic Coach Program are similar to ideas that our respondents suggested for getting organized. These included:

- learning to delegate
- separating work and home time
- increasing time away from work

Another respondent said, "Separate the 'should-do's' from the 'must-do's' and then forget the 'shoulds.' "

**Juggling the Struggle**

Most of our respondents told us that it is time and care for oneself that seems to most often evaporate. It seems so difficult to value time spent on ourselves and to acknowledge the limits of our resources unless illness strikes. Almost half of our respondents said that stresses related to juggling work, family demands, and personal needs led to unhealthy behaviors, such as eating too much, drinking too much alcohol, or giving up regular exercise. We often heard people say with great frustration that, even when they know what they should be doing to manage stress, they can't seem to do these things consistently. This often leads to insomnia, digestive or back problems, heightened anxiety, or other physical problems.

When we are trying to juggle work, home, and self, we are most likely to let the "self-care" ball drop and to sacrifice our own health. A recent Statistics Canada study showed that moving from standard to long working hours was associated with unhealthy weight gain for men, an increase in smoking for both men and women, and an increase in drinking for women. Over time, all of these changes can lead to heart disease and other serious physical problems, as well as an increase in psychological problems such as depression and anxiety, and more marital conflicts and family difficulties. See Chapters 2, 3, and 4 on how to change unhealthy behaviors and strike a better balance in your life.

## Will You Ever Retire?

When it comes to retirement, the experience of respondents in our survey may once again predict some larger trends. According to the majority, the traditional move from all-to-nothing, complete with gold watch and goodbye party, is a thing of the past. Most boomers said they plan to retire gradually – 49 per cent – or not at all – 21 per cent.

A woman in her mid-fifties described how she plans to taper off her work hours in her early sixties while continuing to earn some income. "I always plan to be doing something meaningful," stated a male physician. "I will work as a doctor as long as I can, and I expect I will do more non-remunerative work like teaching and community service as I get older. The important thing for me is to keep my mind active and apply my skills and talents in a useful way."

One woman who is a sister in a religious organization said, "The elder sisters I work with have showed me that, while aging slows you down a little, it certainly does not diminish one's zest for life and ministry. Sisters rarely retire, they just find other ways to minister." Others spoke about changing the nature of their work: for example, switching to independent consulting or turning a pastime such as repairing and troubleshooting with computers into paid work.

When we asked our respondents how they planned to spend their time when retired or partly retired, the answers were varied and creative.

- *More time with family members.* Spending more time with loved ones, particularly with one's partner, was the most frequent response. Those who already had grandchildren talked enthusiastically about the fun they had with them. Those without them said things like "I can't wait for grandchildren" and "I plan to enjoy my kids as adults – and hopefully to have grandchildren."
- *Travel* was high on the list of many – everything from cruising to ecotourism and adventure travel, and volunteering in developing countries.
- *Altruism*, which has been shown to have a positive effect on health, ranks high on the list of retirement goals. Many boomers plan to increase the amount of volunteer work they do. This is often related to their religious faith and will involve helping younger and older

people in the community. Some see official retirement as an opportunity to share their skills in management, budgeting, and training with groups like the United Way and other non-governmental organizations. Others were planning to do things that a hectic work schedule had not allowed. One woman said, "I am going to give blood regularly. I never had time when I was working, and I think it is an important service that we tend to ignore."

• *Lifelong learning and creative pursuits.* Several people talked about returning to school to pursue studies they'd long been interested in or to acquire new skills. Time to pursue creative hobbies such as music, visual arts, and writing was mentioned often. "I want to write a novel, just for fun," said one person. "I have waited a long time to take piano and painting lessons," said another. Others talked about pursuing hobbies such as belly-dancing, quilting, woodworking, singing, bridge, and investing. One woman who was recently diagnosed with cancer spoke passionately about her love for the violin. "I had always thought I would take up fiddling in retirement," she says. "But now I am not waiting until I retire. I have already begun violin lessons, and I love every minute of it."

• *Physical activity.* Many people plan to spend more time being active when they retire, walking, gardening, playing golf, tennis, and skiing. Several spoke wistfully about wanting more time to spend enjoying the outdoors at that particularly Canadian institution, the summer cottage.

## Role Models for Retirement

**Flora MacDonald**, former Canadian cabinet minister and Canada's first woman Minister of Foreign Affairs, is a person who continues to pursue challenge and live life to the fullest as she grows older. She found herself formally "retired" when she was defeated in a federal election at the age of sixty-two. "It was traumatic," she recalls. "After seventeen years in politics, I was suddenly out of a job. In those days, your salary stopped the night you were defeated, and you were expected to vacate your offices within ten days."

Flora's "time off" ended quickly when OXFAM asked her to go as a volunteer to Namibia to monitor troubling pre-election conditions there. "I was immediately immersed in learning about the struggles for democracy in Africa," she says. "I knew I wanted to learn more and contribute more in countries in need around the world."

That first assignment was the beginning of Flora's next career – exciting and important work in human rights, aging, health, and development in many Third World countries. "I am busier now than when I was minister," she says, "and these have been the most exciting twelve years of my life." At seventy-five, she chairs or serves on the boards of twelve national and international organizations. Her work with Future Generations and Care Canada takes her to Afghanistan, Tibet, and other rugged and dangerous countries. "Climbing and sleeping in tents in these severe environments means that I must stay healthy and fit," she notes. Flora eats healthful foods, exercises for an hour every morning, and walks and skates regularly.

Flora has long advocated the removal of all age-limitation policies in the workplace. "I believe that all who are able and want to remain in the formal workplace should do so. To some extent, the demographics of an aging population will force this change. But Canadians in midlife should also consider how they can share their talents in countries that need assistance. Nothing makes me prouder than meeting people in developing countries who tell me how volunteer Canadian engineers, teachers, nurses, and others have helped them establish businesses and infrastructures that have enabled them to move ahead."

While she agrees it is possible to retire from work in a formal sense, Flora does not consider retiring from life an option. "The most important thing one can do in later life is maintain a sense of curiosity. You just don't know how exciting and rewarding life can be after age sixty until you get there!"

**Ramsay Cook**, Canadian historian and retired York University professor, has found balance in retirement – the very thing that most boomers are seeking. He made the decision to retire officially one year earlier than directed by the university. In no way, however, has he retired from life.

"I liked teaching, writing, and research, but toward the end I felt I was repeating myself in the classroom. There was not much innovation or challenge in it for me, so I felt it was time to stop."

When Ramsay first retired, he said yes to everything. "I took on several projects; I was very busy. I guess I was afraid that I would not have anything to do." One of these assignments was serving as a volunteer at Toronto's Daily Food Bank, an activity that he plans to take up again. (See Chapter 11 for more on this.)

Now, after five years of official retirement, Ramsay works about two to three days a week as the general editor of the *Dictionary of Canadian Biography* and as vice president of Associated Medical Services. "It gives me something to do and helps me maintain contact with colleagues, but I can also go away when I want to." For example, he has visited the Galapagos and the Amazon, two places he had always wanted to see. He and his wife continue to travel when they feel like it and to spend time at the cottage near their daughter and her family.

He stays healthy with regular physical activity, including swimming (forty-five minutes four times a week), bicycling, walking, skating, and skiing. "I have been interested in natural history since childhood," says Ramsay, "and I love bird-watching. It kind of gives me a reason to walk."

How has Ramsay Cook found balance in his retirement years? "I was very fortunate that I loved my work before retirement, and I love it now. I still get to do some interesting projects, such as helping out with the recent history series on CBC. I do enough to keep active, but not so much that I get stressed about it."

He also enjoys a very satisfying family life. He and his wife see their two children often and have a new granddaughter, who is their great joy. "I find it hard to understand how people can go to Florida for many months away from their families and children. We are and always were a very close family."

**From the Research**
*Death from Overwork?*
In Japan, a growing number of workers who put in long hours at work have been dying of cardiovascular causes in their most productive years. The Japanese call such a death "Karoshi," which means "death from overwork." Many boomers in Canada and the United States can appreciate this term. Studies show that women who work long hours have a greater chance of

developing depression, and that both men and women who work long hours are more likely to go to the doctor for medical problems than people who work standard hours.

Source: Margot Shields. "Long Working Hours and Health." *Health Reports*. Ottawa: Statistics Canada, Vol. 11, No. 2 (2000).

*Out to Lunch – NOT!*

According to a 2001 survey by the National Restaurant Association in the United States, one of the ways that Americans are working longer is by lunching at their desks. On any given day, some 53 per cent of workers ate at their desks (take-out food, food from vending machines, and food from home) and some 31 per cent of workers skipped lunch altogether. Workers aged fifty-five to sixty-four were least likely to take their full lunch hour.

Source: *University of California at Berkeley Wellness Letter*, Vol. 17, No. 9 (June 2001).

## On the Lighter Side
*Restructuring Experts*

"Restructuring" is a concept that is all too familiar to boomers, as is the tongue-in-cheek story below.

A management restructuring task force was given free tickets to the Montreal Symphony Orchestra. The next day the CEO asked how his employees enjoyed the night. He was handed a memorandum that read:

1. For a considerable period the oboe players had nothing to do. Their number should be reduced and their work spread over the whole orchestra to reduce peaks and troughs in workflow.
2. All twelve violins were playing identical notes. This seems unnecessary duplication, and the section should be drastically downsized.
3. Much effort was involved in playing the demi-semiquavers. This seems excessive refinement, and it is recommended that all notes should be rounded up to the nearest semiquaver. If this were done, it would be possible to use more trainees in the orchestra, and costs would be reduced.

4. No useful purpose is served by repeating with horns the passage that has been handled already by the strings. If all such redundant passages were eliminated, the concert could be reduced from two hours to twenty minutes.

## Questions to Reflect On

Midlife is the time to reassess what is really important in your life and to separate what you really need from what you want. It is critical that you take action to achieve a balance that is good for you, your family, and your work. This means working toward balance as a couple and a family, as well as individually. It is a time to consider retirement options from formal work and to make a plan and commitment to never retire from life.

1. Take some time to reflect on the work that you do – paid and unpaid – and the people you work with. Do your jobs give you satisfaction? If yes, how? If no, what one small change can you make now to help you feel more satisfied about your work?
2. Are you happy with the career you chose to work at for most of your life? Would you like to work at something different? If yes, what can you do now to move toward making that change?
3. When do you plan to retire, if ever? How will you spend your time when you retire? How can you make the time to do some of those things now, rather than wait for retirement?
4. What one small change would enable you to work fewer hours and still meet your financial goals? When will you have this change in place? Who will witness this change?

# CHAPTER EIGHT

# Family First

The family, that dear octopus from whose tentacles we never quite escape, nor in our innermost hearts ever quite wish to.
— Dodie Smith, author, 1896–1990

As mothers and grandmothers, we were not surprised to hear of the joy and satisfaction that family members bring to the midlife men and women who responded to our Healthy Boomer Midlife Survey. It affirmed what we ourselves learned in our research for our first book.

As we explored a little deeper, we noted that family matters were also very challenging in midlife, especially for the sandwich generation, who have teenagers or young children in the home and ailing, aging parents at the same time. Said one woman, "I work full-time, help my mom out, and deal with raging hormones in my teenage daughter and myself . . . all at the same time. I feel a bit like the cheese in a grilled-cheese sandwich."

Relationships of all types, along with our beliefs and values, shape the way we define ourselves as individuals. In midlife, we become more conscious of how important our relationships with family members really are. Losses in midlife, such as children leaving home or the death of a parent, may make us particularly and painfully aware of meaningful relationships. The marriages of our children, the birth of a grandchild, a new romantic relationship or a reconfirmation of an old one may deepen our feeling of being part of a group that surrounds us and holds us with love.

This chapter explores what boomers told us about the complexity and special nature of family relationships, including relations with intimate partners, with children of all ages, and with our aging parents. See Chapter 10 regarding relationships with friends and pets.

**Family Matters**

At midlife, family often means both the family to which we were born – parents, brothers, sisters, etc. – and the family we have created with our partners. These families may or may not include children, grandchildren, and a circle of beloved friends. For midlife women and men on their own, families of choice can extend to nieces and nephews, friends, pets, and voluntary caring relationships with disadvantaged children or isolated seniors. Dr. Elaine Dembe, chiropractor and author of *Passionate Longevity* and *Use the Good Dishes*, says, "I am into 'aunting' in a big way. Mentoring has been so important in my life that I joyfully give to my nephews and now to a grandniece and grandnephews. I get so much pleasure watching them become who they are. Being with little ones allows me to be playful and silly, and that doesn't happen many other places."

Typically, midlife is a time when both men and women reflect on and reevaluate their relationships with their families of origin. Some seek to sort out old hurts and regain closeness with parents and siblings. Some are driven to reconnect with their roots by finding parents they never knew. Others find this too painful or not appropriate.

Most of us know families that carry grudges, sometimes for years. One woman said, "I have an aunt and uncle who have not spoken to each other for years. Now that they are in their eighties they have forgotten why they stopped speaking in the first place, but they carry on this way, regardless. I don't want to feel bitter as I age and cut myself off from my brother or sister. Midlife is the time to let bygones be bygones. It is time to forgive your siblings for things that may have hurt you when you were younger."

To forgive and reconcile may not be possible for everyone, but midlife does give you the opportunity to face the reality of your family situation and work to resolve your unfinished business.

Some midlife women and men make special efforts through family reunions and gatherings to reconnect with siblings, cousins, and other family members on a regular basis. "We started a family reunion when we realized that Mom and Dad may not be here much longer," explained one midlife woman. "The immediate and extended family includes about fifty people. We meet at a designated place every second summer for a three-day weekend and enjoy a variety of events like picnics, a hackers' golf tournament, and dinner at a local community center that we rent for the occasion.

It has brought me closer to my sisters and brother, and allowed my own children to get a sense of how the family works. My parents love it, even though it is noisy and a little crazy sometimes. My father always looks around the room at the family dinner with a satisfied smile and says to my mother, 'And to think that we are responsible for this mob!'"

### Dealing with Family Stress

According to the boomers in our survey, here are the greatest sources of family stress:

- time pressures that make it hard to balance work, intimate relationships, family life, caregiving, and self-care.
- feeling drained of emotional energy: "It is a challenge to give emotional energy to dependents when I have my own emotional challenges, such as menopause, as well as trying to keep my married relationship healthy and deal with pressures at work."
- living away from parents and other older relatives who need support: "My parents live four hundred miles away and one of them is very ill. I call daily and drive up to see them most weekends. This takes a lot of physical and emotional energy, and I am away from my own family a lot."
- financial pressures: "We chose to live in a safe, clean neighborhood with good schools and recreation facilities, but the cost is high; we struggle with constantly feeling poor."
- social pressures: "We try to ignore the constant pressures to 'keep up with the Joneses.' My husband works part-time to ensure the children get real time with their parents."
- competing priorities: "I want to go back to school, but I need to get my children through university before my organization 'retires' me."
- unresolved conflicts between family members: "My partner and her mother have never gotten along. It seems much worse now that her mother is elderly and she is in menopause. It affects our whole family."

When asked how they deal with family stress, respondents repeatedly cited the need to keep communication channels open and deal with things before tensions build up. For example, people suggested "having regular chats at the dinner table to find out what is going on in everyone's life" and "being interested when things are going well and not just when there are problems." One woman said, "It is also important to clearly let children know what is expected of them and what they can expect from you."

Respondents suggested the following strategies to deal with conflict:

- Openly state that there is a problem and agree to sit down and talk about it.
- Stress the process – talking it out in an honest way – rather than the outcome.
- Be tolerant and try to understand other people's positions.
- Work toward finding mutually agreed-upon solutions that everyone can accept. One man said, "We ask our kids if they can 'live with' a certain solution, even if it is not perfect. Usually they can."

Sometimes these suggestions are easier said than done. Because of the complexities in family relations, putting these strategies into practice can be a daunting task. "I try not to get discouraged when things don't work out," said one woman. "Emotions run high with teenagers in the house, and sometimes we just aren't able to talk things out. I think this is normal in most families and that people should not feel bad if they cannot always find solutions. As long as we continue to love and respect each other, it will work out in the end."

## Intimate Relationships

Positive relations with our partners are critical to our well-being, yet they tend to be the ones that absorb the bulk of our stress in midlife. We pull it together for our kids, we look after our parents when they need extra care, we fulfil our work commitments. But too often our intimate relationships don't get much more nurturing than we do. In North America, most boomers – 80 per cent – are married or living common-law. Many of these are second or third live-in relationships that often lead to the blending of two families and a complicated variety of joint and solo parenting arrangements. "My husband and I feel like an anomaly," said one fifty-four-year-old woman. "We've been married for twenty-eight years, and none of our friends have been together nearly that long."

The majority of respondents to the Healthy Boomer Midlife Survey told us that they were satisfied (41%) or "somewhat satisfied" (24%) with their intimate relationships. Yet they were also clear that midlife partnerships face numerous challenges and changes that can threaten their stability.

The most common issues that plague family life in general were lack of time and not enough energy to nurture relationships. Boomers told us that there was "too much routine and not enough quality time." One man observed how difficult it is to maintain some level of intimacy when "95 per cent of our communication is operational, about scheduling, kids, chores and responsibilities." Another person said, "With two careers, kids, and daily stresses, there is very little time together and only rare moments of intimacy."

Some spoke about how personal emotional problems interfered with intimacy. One said, "My own fears and anxiety about aging and becoming disabled get in the way." Another said that financial pressures, combined with depression, prevented her and her partner from having a satisfying intimate relationship. Others recognized that hormonal mood swings, general irritability, and impatience took their toll.

One midlife woman said, "I am disappointed in our midlife relation-ship, because my husband's health has deteriorated to the point he is unable to do much with me." Several cited a spouse's drinking as a major problem.

When we asked what were the major roadblocks to communication, these were some of the answers:

- not enough listening on both sides;
- not enough shared interests;
- Mars and Venus – men and women worrying about different things;
- an unwillingness to take emotional risks with each other;
- avoiding intimate conversation.

## SOME HIGHLIGHTS FROM THE HEALTHY
## BOOMER MIDLIFE SURVEY

| *How satisfied are you with your current intimate relationship?* | |
|---|---|
| Very satisfied | 41% |
| Somewhat satisfied | 24% |
| Neither satisfied nor dissatisfied | 7% |
| Somewhat dissatisfied | 1% |
| Very dissatisfied | 5% |
| Not applicable/No answer | 22% |

### Better in Midlife

We also asked boomers, "What is more fulfilling about your relationship in midlife than when you were younger?" Their responses were heartening.

Many spoke of their greater maturity and their partners' maturity as positive factors. As one man put it, "I am more mature. I know myself better. I'm able to give more and not sweat the small stuff." Another said, "We have the maturity to overlook minor aggravations." A midlife woman said, "I am a stronger person. I know what I want and don't want, and I am not afraid to ask for it."

In addition to greater self-assurance, respondents of both sexes noted a kinder and more realistic assessment and appreciation of their partners. They said such things as:

- "We are accepting of each other – faults, annoyances, and all. We are what we are, and we both accept that. When we were younger, we both got annoyed and tried to change the other."
- "We are both very comfortable with each other, like a pair of old shoes."
- "I look at this person as a human being and know that neither of us is perfect. I accept him for who he is."

Others spoke of the importance of shared history. "We have been through everything together," said one woman. "We have shared the joys of growing children and now we have beautiful grandchildren. It is a deep part of our bond."

The ability to communicate more openly in midlife was a plus for some boomer couples, compared to their earlier years. "We have more confidence in each other and in our relationship," said one woman. A man noted, "We are more open and more skilled in communicating." According to a fifty-five-year-old woman, "Now we seem to be able to solve most problems ourselves. We work to communicate clearly and supportively. We love each other more as time goes on. It has taken effort to achieve this in our work-stressed lives."

Most respondents observed that understanding, trust, and friendship more than compensated for reduced excitement and spontaneity in midlife. One said, "Our relationship is much more fulfilling: we laugh, we really enjoy each other." Another said, "I take nothing for granted. I feel very grateful for all the richness in my life."

Not all successful midlife relationships happen under the same roof. There is a growing trend among older boomers with a certain level of financial comfort and grown children to be committed to each other but to maintain separate residences. A fifty-nine-year-old woman said, "My partner and I met a long time after our first marriages had ended. Our kids were in college or on their own. We tried living together and it was a disaster, but we still really loved each other. Finally, we realized we could stay together better by each having some space that was totally our own. It's not ideal, but it works for us."

*When Marriage Fails*

The positive dimensions of relationships discussed above do not always happen the first time around. As is the case with so many other current social mores, the boomers are the first generation to make divorce and remarriage or common-law cohabitation everyday occurrences. Divorce rates in Canada doubled between 1971 and 1982 and hit an all-time high in 1987, when the first wave of boomers were in their mid-thirties. Since then, those rates have declined steadily. However, this does not necessarily mean that marriages are more stable than they were in the 1980s. It may instead reflect the growing trend, among people of all age groups, to live together in common-law relationships.

Despite the greater number of common-law unions, most midlife men and women still opt for legal marriage. In the Healthy Boomer Midlife

Survey, 47 per cent of people were still in their first marriages, while 19 per cent were in their second partnerships and 11 per cent in their third or beyond. Many boomers have learned painful lessons in early relationships that they hope will help them make happier and more secure choices in their midlife marriages.

Forty-four-year-old **Lindsay** is getting married this summer – for the fourth time. After her first marriage, to her high-school sweetheart, didn't work out, she married a man who "seemed to be smart and loyal and very different" from her first husband. They had two children together. But when husband number two had an affair and then left her for the other woman, Lindsay was devastated. She rushed into a third midlife marriage.

She says now, "I knew in my heart and my guts that this was a mistake, that I should have waited, but I let fear, loneliness, and lust get in the way. Marrying my third husband was a way to avoid facing the black hole of my depression and my feelings of failure and grief over losing my dream of a happy, intact family." He turned out to be an alcoholic and a compulsive gambler. The marriage lasted less than a year.

At this point, Lindsay realized that there was a pattern to her relationships that she was in danger of repeating again. She recognized that she needed help to understand what she was doing and how to change it. She joined a weekly group-therapy program that she has attended for the past three years. She describes her experience: "It is not an easy process, but eventually I saw how physical attraction clouds my vision and that 'romance' is not the same thing as love. I finally figured out that all my good intentions to rescue a man will not change him into the man of my fantasies. So I had better look for someone I like, rather than trying to change some attractive guy into someone I can like. I realized that I have many other sources of love and support in my life, such as family members and friends. I learned that I can have a healthy family life without a partner by my side."

We asked Lindsay how she and her future husband plan to make their marriage work. "First of all," she said, "we accept and love each other for who we are. I am committed to continuing to work on my issues in therapy. And if things in our relationship are really getting to me, I will work hard not to keep my feelings bottled up inside." She and her husband will have three children in their new blended family. They have made a commitment to seek outside help if difficulties arise.

When marriages fail, many people suffer. One woman describes how sad she felt when her ex-partner's bitterness about their divorce pushed her in-laws to take sides and to cut off contact with her after thirteen years of a very close relationship. "It all changed when my ex-mother-in-law was dying. I went to her and she welcomed me back as a friend. I attended the funeral with her family and my ex-husband's new family. We cried together. Now, I stay in touch with my ex-husband's siblings and the old wounds have healed. This gives me a sense of peace, a feeling that some important unfinished business has been dealt with. It is also good for my children, because the tension is gone for them. They sense a difference and find it easier to talk about me with my ex-husband's family."

In our practices we are also finding that the young adult children of divorced families often have their own difficulties in relationships. Some are very fearful of committed relationships; others enter into serious relationships very quickly and are reluctant to let go. How significant this trend is remains to be seen.

### Recovering from Broken Trust

Some people shared their stories of working to heal painful breaches of trust within their relationships. Her youngest daughter was two when **Janet** discovered that her husband was having an affair with another woman who was a close family friend. While things were very rocky for a while, they managed to work through this and they have a solid marriage now, ten years later. Janet credits this to the fact that they both took responsibility for what happened and that they both worked hard to make the relationship work. This meant adjusting their attitudes toward each other and accepting that there were things they didn't like about each other, and that those things weren't going to change. Janet says that the couples counseling they had was "immensely important." "We were fortunate to have a gifted therapist who tuned into both of us and helped us build on the strengths of our relationship." They set goals for the future and focused on them, instead of on the "rather icky" recent past. Janet adds, "For me, one of the most important factors was leaving the home and neighborhood where this all happened, so that we had a bit of a fresh start. Even ten years later, there is a lot of forgiveness on both sides but we are not at a point of laughing about it. Maybe we never will be, and maybe keeping it in a solemn place will remind us of the pain we worked through."

### Peers' Advice about Intimate Relationships

We asked boomer couples what they do to promote positive communication in their day-to-day lives. The majority emphasized the necessity of making the commitment to talk with each other, whether it was over dinner, while walking, while having a cup of tea, or after the kids were in bed. One man said, "It won't just happen. You have to make it a priority and you have to make a habit of it." This is what others told us:

- "We try to talk things over and listen to each other's opinions whether we agree or not."
- "We try to be less reactive in tense situations."
- "We take time to talk, go for walks, cuddle a lot, and go on one short vacation each year without the kids."
- "We work on projects and plan specific activities together."
- "We like each other, and we laugh a lot."
- "We go to couples therapy when we need to."
- "We discuss problems and don't harbor grudges."
- "We validate and acknowledge each other's point of view."

### Intergenerational Wisdom

We asked our respondents to tell us the most important piece of advice they would give to their children or young friends about making relationships work. Not surprisingly, they talked about the basics of kindness, respect, a sense of humor, and talking to each other. In addition, one fifty-six-year-old mother and grandmother gave this advice: "Always keep this question in the back of your mind: Will I have regrets if I make this decision about our relationship or treat my spouse a certain way?" Several emphasized the importance of pursuing your own goals and maintaining independence. One person listed three important components of a healthy relationship: communication, commitment, and common sense. Another very important bit of advice was "Don't forget to hug your partner, and never stop whispering 'I love you' in his or her ear!"

Just as boomers offer sage advice about intimate relationships to give to their own children, we have a lot to learn from the generation that came before us. We talked with the author, feminist, and social activist **June Callwood** about her fifty-eight-year marriage to Trent Frayne, and asked what advice she would give to boomers.

June said that when she sees young people leaving relationships and starting new ones, she feels concerned about how easy they think it is for them and their children to separate and start over. "There is little appreciation that perfection is not possible," she says. "They think the next one will be 'it.' But relationships are hard work. Even after fifty-eight years, we both continue to make small compromises."

She explained that many of her peers in long-term relationships continue to "plod on during their seventies and eighties, through thin and thinner." "But," she says, "there is a big payback. When you become frail, there is someone who knows you to the ground. I don't know if someone who has been with you for only fifteen years and grew up believing that if a relationship isn't perfect, it is okay to just leave it will really want to stick around when an illness like Alzheimer disease happens. Old age is a very good time to have someone around . . ."

June says that the thinnest time for her and her husband was about fifteen years into the marriage. "We were bored with each other, but we got through that. Despite the fact that we are very different, we have learned how to stay together. My husband is eighty-four and had a frail winter, but I just can't imagine life without him. That's kind of a nice feeling."

She added: "We are also aware how very good it is for our adult children and grandchildren that we are still together. I really like the continuity and feel a lot of pleasure knowing that this part of my life is uncomplicated."

### For the Love of Children

When we asked our survey respondents what gives them most joy in life, their love for their children was the most frequent answer. Watching their offspring grow and thrive and "turn into responsible adults" was a common answer. "Seeing my daughter finish college was one of the greatest joys of my life," said one forty-four-year-old woman.

Another woman described her anxiety about seeing her last child go away to university. "We were so close. We talked every day. I was afraid there would be a big hole in my life that I wouldn't be able to fill. A friend told me to relax and break out the champagne. She joked that there would be gas in the car and food in the refrigerator after he left. Four weeks after he was gone, I realized that our relationship had not ended, just changed. We still talked on the phone. The trust we had established grew instead of diminishing. He was more understanding and grateful now that he lived on his own. So I phoned my friend and said, 'You were right. Crack open the bottle of champagne. I'll be right over.'"

Many of the respondents to the Healthy Boomer Midlife Survey talked about how much they looked forward to being grandparents. Those who already had grandchildren talked repeatedly about how satisfied and happy they were in that relationship. "My children get upset when I tell them that grandmothering is a lot more fun than parenting," said one woman. "My grandkids and had a great time reading *Harry Potter* together. They voted me 'Best Grandma in the World' when I took them out of school to go and see the movie. I never could have done that with my own kids. I was too busy and too concerned about their school marks. The beauty of being a grandparent is that you don't have twenty-four-hour responsibility. You can love and indulge them, give them all your attention, and wear everybody out having fun. You don't even have to wash their clothes. You can send them home exhausted, happy, and dirty."

Several women who do not have children of their own talked about the importance and fun of being an aunt. "Being an aunt or uncle is a lot like being a grandparent," explained a woman who corresponds with her young niece weekly by e-mail and postcard. "We have a special relationship. She can talk with me about things she can't tell her mom or dad. I introduce her to new restaurants and take her skating and bike riding when we get together. My relationship with her is a highlight of my life."

### Young Families in Midlife

Boomers are unique in the wide variation of their ages when they have taken on parenting roles. Indeed, although we three authors of this book are all in our fifties, one of us is a grandmother of seven, one is the mother of two young people in their early twenties, and one is the mother of a five-year-old. Choosing to be parents later in life than was the norm for our parents' generation sometimes happens because of longer stays in school, later marriages, and second relationships, and sometimes because boomer women decided to establish their careers or businesses before having children.

**Kathryn** and **Dianne** adopted two children when they were ages thirty-seven and forty-two, respectively. Dianne explains that becoming parents in midlife was not a conscious decision to wait until they were older. "Both of us always knew we wanted to have children," says Dianne, "but circumstances delayed things. I went back to school and started a business. After we knew our relationship was what we wanted it to be, we spent a number of years trying to get pregnant. When that didn't work, we settled on adoption. By then I was forty."

Kathryn and Dianne's children were two and a half and three and a half years old when they joined the family. "We talked a lot about the implications of being older parents," said Kathryn, "for example, knowing that our kids would be going to university when we were in our sixties. So in some ways, the idea of adopting children who were a little older was appealing. We tried to prepare ourselves, but I don't think anyone can be really ready for going from being child-free to having two active toddlers in the house from one day to the next."

Both made big adjustments in their careers to accommodate their new roles. Kathryn works four days a week outside the home and spends Fridays helping at the school, taking the children to appointments, and doing household errands. Dianne went from full-time to half-time consulting, but now that the children are aged seven and eight she works four days a week. "At age forty-seven," she says, "I am aware that I am at the height of my earning and learning power. I am anxious to get back to full-time work."

"All the activity with the children helps to keep us feeling young," says Dianne, "but I admit that I feel tired a lot. It feels strange, too, when I go to the school and most of the other parents are in their twenties and thirties. Sometimes I feel like I could be their mother." There is also the matter of dealing with older parents who are ill while raising young children. For example, Dianne needed to spend seven weeks with her mother before her death, leaving Kathryn to hold the fort at home. Between parenting, work, and other midlife responsibilities, time is at a premium. "We have stayed close and used all of our problem-solving skills to keep our relationship strong and be good parents at the same time," says Dianne.

"There are pros and cons to taking on a parenting role in midlife," says

Kathryn, "but I believe in living the life you have and enjoying it to the fullest. I think we are more confident in the parenting role because of our age and experience. I regret that our children do not have two sets of grandparents like I did as a kid, and that they will likely be in their forties when we die. But we are so blessed to have them."

*Life with Teenagers*

Like generations of parents before us, numerous people talked about the challenges of parenting teenagers, especially at the busiest time of their careers, and often with the added responsibility of aging parents. "Between work, handling two teenagers, and driving to Montreal to be with my mother and her sister, there is not much time or energy left for an intimate relationship with my wife," said one man.

**Nancy** has two daughters, aged sixteen and thirteen, and a sixteen-year-old "surrogate son" from the neighborhood, who spends a lot of time with them. She says that, with kids, it's important to check in when things are going well and not just when they are not, even though finding and making time for this is a challenge. "I think it helps that I am genuinely interested in their friends and what everyone is doing." She adds, "And it keeps me young."

When we asked her how she balances parenting teens with a full-time job, she laughed and said, "That's the million-dollar question!" It helps that her husband is very involved with their daughters, and one of them has always managed to have a job near home. As much as possible, they have dinner together with the television off, so they can talk. She also uses a "sitting on the end of the bed" strategy that she says is very helpful. She'll knock on their doors to ask a practical question or get something and then just "kind of hang out" for a while. This often allows meaningful exchanges to happen that might not come about otherwise.

In terms of advice to parents with teens, Nancy says, "The first words that come to my mind are 'fairness for both.' I tell the girls that this is new to us and that we're on a steep learning curve. We are doing our best. At the same time, I want them to tell us if they feel we're being overbearing or too strict." Nancy and her husband's style of parenting calls for lots of negotiating around rules that the girls can now joke about.

The next important word for Nancy is "connectedness." She says, "One major reward of dedicating time to connecting with kids is an open and honest relationship based on caring and affection. I spend a lot of time creating opportunities for connecting, such as outings to the theater, or skiing for a few days, in order to have family times on a regular basis. But I always try to be aware that, as the kids grow, so must our tolerance for their increasing independence."

*Fathers Parenting More*

Margaret Mead once said that "the supreme test of any civilization is whether it can socialize men by teaching them to be fathers." Yet most boomers were raised with role models who believed their chief contribution to the family should be a financial – not a caring – one. Their own fathers were more emotionally distant than they would have liked. In midlife, many men become more conscious of their desire to be more involved in caring roles. Increasingly, midlife men are contributing time and energy to the care of their children, grandchildren, and aging parents. For some men, becoming parents a second time around allows them to deal with their grief over what they missed the first time, as well as to experience the joy and magic of young children. One said, "I feel so blessed to be able to really be a parent this time. It helps me be a better father to my grown-up children as well."

## The Challenges of Caregiving

Although a caregiver can be a spouse, child, parent, friend, or neighbor, most often it is a woman. A typical caregiver for older people is age forty-five to fifty-five, female, married, and employed outside the home. She can expect to spend as many years caring for a parent as she does for her children. There is also a good chance that she will be a caregiver to more than one person during her lifetime. Because many women are marrying and having children later, they frequently find themselves in the sandwich generation, caring for their children and parents at the same time.

In the Healthy Boomer Midlife Survey, 43 per cent of women and 21 per cent of men were providing some form of support to an older or disabled relative. Most caregivers spent up to ten hours per week caring for older people, although 21 per cent of the men and 23 per cent of the women spent more than thirty hours – the equivalent of a full-time job. Generally, the more ill an older person is, the more time he or she needs in care. While twice as many women as men were serving in caregiving roles, those men who were involved spent significant amounts of time supporting older relatives.

Most were providing emotional support and company to older people; almost one-quarter of these also assisted with housework, meals, and home maintenance. Other activities included helping parents with financial concerns – such as investing and paying bills – assisting with transportation and shopping, and arranging for nursing care and home help.

## SOME HIGHLIGHTS FROM THE HEALTHY BOOMER MIDLIFE SURVEY

*Do you provide support to older or disabled relatives who do not live with you?*

|  | Men | Women |
|---|---|---|
| No | 79% | 57% |
| Yes | 21% | 43% |

*How many hours do you spend caring for children, older relatives, or disabled family members?*

|  | Men | Women |
|---|---|---|
| More than 30 hours per week | 15% | 23% |
| Between 10 and 30 hours per week | 31% | 19% |
| Between 5 and 10 hours per week | 14% | 14% |
| Between 1 and 5 hours per week | 26% | 30% |
| Less than 1 hour per week | 14% | 14% |

*How do you care for older or disabled relatives (more than one answer is possible)?*

| | |
|---|---|
| Provide emotional support and company | 46% |
| Help with housework and home maintenance | 23% |
| Help with meals | 23% |
| Take care of finances, such as investing, paying bills | 15% |
| Help with transportation and shopping | 8% |
| Arrange for nursing care and home help | 8% |
| Other | 8% |

*The Gains of Caregiving*

**Tom** explains how he reestablished a caring relationship with his parents after they became sick. "When I moved to Toronto, I did not see them that often. That all changed when my father had a major stroke. It is very hard to connect with him now because he cannot walk, talk, or feed himself. There are days when he does not react at all, but then the next day he smiles and is obviously happy to see me. It is very different with my mother. She has serious heart disease and is quite frail, but our relationship has grown much closer again. On the one hand, I am still her child, and she still treats me as such sometimes. On the other hand, I see her as quite vulnerable now. I admire how she copes physically and emotionally. She goes to the hospital twice a day to feed my father. My sister and I had to help her with selling her house and teach her about all the things my father always did, such as how to handle finances and insurance issues. But she is learning. Now, in her old age, she is establishing her own identity, not just one that came via my father."

Tom drives four to five hours each way to spend every second weekend with his mother. "At first I felt like I was walking on eggs around her. But now that I spend more time with her, we can discuss anything – even what will happen with my father or could happen to her. The other benefit is that I have been able to review her whole life history with her – to hear about her youth, her marriage to my father, my own birth, and growing up with my sister. If my parents had not become sick, I would never have had the chance to hear these stories and have this much time with my mother.

"We get along well on these weekends. I know her routine and I am out of my routine, so I just adjust to hers. I don't try to change or correct her. I am just with her. I am not sure if we would get on each other's nerves if I were there for longer than a weekend. But for now, we have developed a long-distance relationship that really works."

*The Many Factors Affecting Our Experience of Caregiving*

The first factor underlying our caregiving roles is the nature of the relationship and experiences we had with our parents in the past. As one woman described her situation, "No matter what I do, my mom is never happy. She stopped living one day more than twenty years ago, when the police came to our door to tell her that her only son, my brother, had died in a motorcycle accident. From then on, it was as if we, my sister and I, did not exist or matter. I knew she loved us, but our family was never the same. For a while, she found a bit of comfort while she was looking after my dad, who had dementia. When he passed on, her 'purpose' was gone too. She is always unwell, unhappy. No matter what my sister and I try to do for her, it never works."

The second factor is the older person's own ability to deal with change and growing dependence. One woman described her surprise and pleasure about her mother's adjustment to moving to a nursing home. "I always worried about how my mother would deal with her disabilities. I was very nervous the first time I went to see her, after my brother had moved her to a seniors' residence with nursing care. To all of our surprise, she loved the companionship she found at the residence, compared to the long days alone at my brother's home. Within a short time she started to enjoy singing groups. She took up painting and referred to her own art with the same pride as if she had created a masterpiece. Because of her positive attitude, she gets a lot of visitors. Her children, grandchildren, and great-grandchildren all love to go and see her."

A third factor that seems to be a particular problem in midlife is the amount of available time one has to expend in caregiving. This is especially true for the sandwich generation.

"Having children in midlife keeps you young but busy," said a fifty-one-year-old woman. "My son has learning disabilities and he is doing really well now that we have discovered it. My mother has Alzheimer's. Even though she is in a home, I need to go and visit her three times a week. But this is better than trying to manage at home. She has a boyfriend at the home, and that is a real plus for her and me!"

"My parents could use more of my time," said one man, "but I can't find any extra to give. The reward is the actual time we do spend together." One midlife woman said, "The challenges are time and fatigue, as well as being 'up' and accepting of the situation. It is important to be a positive, upbeat companion, but this can be extremely hard at times. I have grown a lot closer to my dad and learned a lot about his childhood and mine. He is a very funny man!"

A fourth factor in one's experience of caregiving with older people is our own comfort level with the end of life. The boomer generation's denial of the reality of death and our failure to see it as a natural progression inhibit us in helping our aging parents deal with their own decline and progressive illness. (See Chapter 12 for more on this subject.)

Of course, some people make the best preparations possible for an inevitable death. Dr. Lhotsky recalls one case in which she was attending a patient's mother at home while she was dying. "The old woman's daughter was a palliative-care nurse who took time off work to look after her mother. She moved her mother into her own home, put the bed in their living room, and stayed with her until she died. It was peaceful and loving. She and her mother were as comfortable as you can be with the dying process. They saw it as the final passage in her mother's full life."

*Caring for the Caregiver*

Most often, adult children strive to help their older parents live independently at home for as long as possible. Their parents' need for day-to-day help with household duties and personal care gradually increases. Sometimes difficult behaviors associated with illness and frustration become hard to handle. It is often difficult to get and maintain home care and other support services. Over time, the caregivers' stamina is depleted, and sometimes they are forced to give up work or time spent with other family members to continue providing that support.

"Two years ago I was helping to care for all four parents," said one fifty-five-year-old woman. "At the time, I thought the challenge was not enough hours in the day. I now realize it was my guilt for not being superhuman enough to handle it all, and feeling angry sometimes because I had this added responsibility." Another woman in her early forties said, "I ask myself how much I am doing out of expectation and obligation. I am still struggling to work through this."

Some of our respondents talked about the need to care for themselves, or else both people in the relationship suffer. One woman said, "My salvation is Sunday morning in bed with a hot cup of tea, a newspaper, and a Do Not Disturb sign. A cooperative family helps!"

Sharing the load is critical for successful caregivers. One fifty-five-year-old woman said, "We have a very close, large family, and we share the joys, sorrows, and helping activities related to our parents' conditions." Children who live in the same city or town as their parents tend to take on the primary caregiving roles. Others talked about the importance of hired helpers – such as cleaning services and paid sitters – and community services such as homecare and Meals on Wheels.

## From the Research
*More Care Equals More Stress*
According to the 1996 Canadian General Social Survey, those caregivers who spend the most time providing care to older people suffer the highest level of psychological and emotional stress. Most women (83%) and men (89%) who spent 7.5 hours or more per week helping seniors reported some level of stress. This level rose with each additional hour. Some 45 per cent of the women and 54 per cent of the men reported changes and restrictions on their own social activities, holiday plans, finances, and sleep patterns because they provided at least 7.5 hours of this care each week.

On the other hand, in a recent study of caregivers, virtually all could identify positive aspects of caregiving, including companionship, fulfillment, enjoyment, and the satisfaction of meeting an obligation and helping to improve someone else's quality of life.

Source: Frederick, J. A., and J. E. Fast. "Eldercare in Canada: Who Does How Much?" *Canadian Social Trends* (Autumn 1999); and Cohen, C., A. Colantonio, and L. Vernich. *International Journal of Geriatric Psychiatry* (February 2002).

## On the Lighter Side
*Kids on Marriage*
Q. *Who should you marry?*
A. "You got to find somebody who likes the same stuff. Like, if you like sports, she should like it that you like sports, and she should keep the chips and dip coming."

Alan, age 10

Q. *What is the right age to get married?*
A. "Twenty-three is the best age, because you know the person *forever* by then."

Camille, age 10

Q. *How can a stranger tell if two people are married?*
A. "Married people usually look happy to talk to other people."
   Eddie, age 6

Q. *Is it better to be single or married?*
A. "I don't know which is better, but I'll tell you one thing. I'm never going to have sex with my wife. I don't want to be all grossed out."
   Theodore, age 8

Q. *How would the world be different if people didn't get married?*
A. "There sure would be a lot of kids to explain, wouldn't there?"
   Kelvin, age 8

Q. *How would you make a marriage work?*
A. "Tell your wife that she looks pretty even if she looks like a truck."
   Ricky, age 10

**Questions to Reflect On**
Midlife is a time to appreciate the importance of family – both those to which we were born and those we have created. Respect, love, communication, and taking time are key ingredients in healthy relationships with partners, parents, children, and other family members.

1. When is the last time you "checked in" with the family members with whom you live? What day next week will you sit down together and do so?
2. What is one fun thing you've been putting off doing with your children or grandchildren? Set a date to do it.
3. What are three things you appreciate about your partner? Make a point of telling him or her.
4. What is one of your favorite activities to do with your partner? Set a specific date to do it.
5. What is one loving thing you could comfortably say or do with your parents, or in their memory?
6. If you are a caregiver who is feeling exhausted or resentful, do you honestly believe that you must do as much as you are doing now?

If not, who can you ask for help (or hire) and what specifically will you ask them to do? Is there a family member you can call on to give you a break? Could your loved one go to a respite program in the community to help you regain your energy?

7. As a caregiver, what is one nurturing thing you can do for yourself this week to help you feel rejuvenated (walk, meditate, find time to read, go to a movie, etc.)?

# CHAPTER NINE

# *Better Sex in Midlife*

If sex is such a natural phenomenon, how come there are so many books on how to do it?

— Bette Midler

Twenty-five hundred years ago, Socrates believed that being freed from the responsibility of having sex was one of the good things about growing older. When asked if he still had intercourse with women, he answered, "Most joyfully did I escape it, as though I had run away from a sort of frenzied and savage monster." For many boomers, the opposite extreme seems to be the case. Having sex into old age is seen as normal and healthy – something we feel entitled to. If our sexual desire wanes or if we choose not to have sex regularly, we wonder if there is something wrong with us. The reality probably lies somewhere in between.

## Better Sex?

The boomer generation has seen a virtual revolution in outward attitudes toward sex. Most North American boomers lived through the "free love" movement of the 1960s and 1970s, saw nudity come to the mainstream American stage (in the musical *Hair*), attended consciousness-raising groups on human sexuality, and listened to more and more explicit music about sex. Many of us have laughed with Eve Ensler's *Vagina Monologues* and Sally's on-screen imitation of an orgasm in *When Harry Met Sally*. But while most boomers can comfortably talk about sex outside the bedroom, we continue to hear in our clinic that, inside the bedroom, talking about sex – and the problems related to sex and desire – is still not easy. In midlife, a host of things can get in the way of satisfying sex. These include physical changes related to aging and menopause, psychological issues such as depression, stress, and unresolved feelings from the past, boredom, overwork, fatigue, and unresolved negative feelings toward one's partner. Men and women who return to dating after the breakup of long-term relationships face some new and frightening aspects of sex in the twenty-first century, including the need to protect themselves from HIV/AIDS and other sexually transmitted diseases.

Happily, many of the people we surveyed reported that sex is better in midlife than it was when they were younger. They cited closeness, tenderness, trust, pleasure, and security in knowing their partners over time. "Sex is comfortable, more satisfying, *yummy* when it happens," said one boomer. "Lovemaking is more sensitive and it lasts longer," explained another.

Others said they were not as shy about saying what they needed and not as worried about the outcomes:

- "I can speak with more courage now about what I want, first to myself and then to my partner."
- "When I was younger I was self-conscious and afraid. Now I have come to see myself as a passionate, sexual being."
- "I am more relaxed, knowing there is less risk of pregnancy and no babies in the way. What a relief to be through with that!"
- "I have less performance anxiety. If I do not climax, it is no big deal."
- "It's okay if we are too tired and fall asleep."

Humor and better communication were mentioned often as key factors that make sex better in midlife. Said one man, "If it does not work, we laugh, make jokes, and talk about how we will improve it the next time."

### SOME HIGHLIGHTS FROM THE HEALTHY BOOMER MIDLIFE SURVEY

| *Do you have a fulfilling sexual relationship?* | | |
|---|---|---|
| | Men | Women |
| Always | 17% | 11% |
| Most of the time | 50% | 36% |
| Some of the time | 28% | 42% |
| Never | 5% | 11% |

| | |
|---|---|
| Women who said they have less interest in sex: | 39% |
| Men who said their female partners have less interest in sex: | 33% |

| | |
|---|---|
| Men who said they have less interest in sex: | 25% |
| Women who said their male partners have less interest in sex: | 26% |

### When Desire Wanes

While sex can be more satisfying in midlife, it can be challenging and difficult, too. When asked what was better about sex in midlife, one woman replied, "Are you kidding? Well, okay . . . he is not getting up to go home after sex is over."

According to our survey, women and men in midlife "read" each other pretty well. Some 25 per cent of men said that they had less interest in sex; 26 per cent of women said their male partners were less interested. More women than men – 39 per cent – said they were less interested in sex in midlife themselves; 33 per cent of men said that their female partners were less interested.

Fifty per cent of our male respondents claimed to have fulfilling sexual relationships "most of the time" compared to 36 per cent of women. Men were more likely than women to "always" have fulfilling sexual relationships (17% versus 11%). Women were twice as likely as men to "never" have fulfilling sexual relationships, but interestingly women were twice as likely as men to report fulfillment "some of the time." Those who never had a fulfilling sexual relationship were small in number for both men and women, with the women saying "never" twice as many times.

Two related factors – fatigue and a lack of time for sex and intimacy – were most often identified as the greatest challenges to satisfying sex in midlife. "I work ten to twelve hours a day, so I often lack the energy to be spontaneous," said one man. Another said, "When you have no time for sex on a regular basis, it turns into a habit of just doing without."

One woman described how she and her partner used the macabre in a humorous way to let each other know when they were just too tired to engage. After reading about "necrophilia" (making love to a dead person), she started using the word as code for "Not tonight, dear, I'm too tired . . ."

Different levels of desire were the next-most-common problem in sexual relationships. "My libido is a lot lower than my husband's," said one woman, "so we have difficulties satisfying both of us no matter what we do." Another woman described a compromise she and her husband had agreed to in order to deal with this problem. "We have agreed to have sex twice a week – on Tuesdays and Fridays. This way he knows we will make love twice a week and I know it will *not* be five times a week. This seems to work fairly well for us."

Other people talked about differences in arousal, erection difficulties, and menopause problems such as a dry vagina and mood swings. Some had lost interest in their partners. Others were unhappy with their bodies ("I feel fat and less than sexy or attractive") or with their partners' bodies ("My sexual relationship with my husband has deteriorated in the last five years due to his poor health and obesity.")

Those who are on their own talked about not having a sexual partner and how hard it is to find a meaningful sexual relationship when you are single or divorced. Lacking a partner is a very common experience as we grow older, especially for women. Lee Stones, an expert in sexuality and aging, tells woman who live alone "to get out there and buy a good vibrator." When she says this, women nod their heads in appreciation. The need for a healthy sex life when one is alone is rarely acknowledged, let alone talked about.

It has always been common for older men to partner with younger women. Now, increasingly, boomer women have been breaking traditional taboos themselves. We have watched celebrities such as actors Mary Tyler Moore, Carol Burnett, rock star Patti Smith, and former Prime Minister Kim Campbell become involved with younger men.

### When the Physical Gets in the Way

Numerous physical conditions can cause sexual problems in midlife. For men in midlife, the incidence of erectile dysfunction (ED) starts to increase. Chronic illness, depression, and the use of antidepressants or other drugs, such as those prescribed for hypertension and high cholesterol levels, can interfere with erections. Recreational drugs such as alcohol can also cause ED. Sometimes, changing the type of medication or decreasing one's alcohol intake can reduce ED.

Viagra (sildenafil) has proven itself an important solution when there are physical reasons for impotence. It helps men whose erections are not firm enough to engage in intercourse and enables those who may have no erections at all to have normal intercourse. Viagra works in about 70 per cent of cases of persistent ED, although men with heart conditions who take nitrate drugs cannot use "the little blue pill." The combination can trigger an extreme drop in blood pressure that could be fatal.

The most common complaint we hear from women is low sexual desire. Like erectile dysfunction in men, this can result from physical or psychological causes or sometimes a combination of both. Many women who suffer from vaginal dryness and therefore discomfort during intercourse use different forms of hormone replacement therapy (HRT) and/or specific lubricants. For those who have had both ovaries removed or who suffer from a clinical testosterone deficiency, testosterone replacement usually proves helpful. However, testosterone is not a panacea. When low levels of desire are related to other factors, such as problems in the relationship, hormones are not a quick fix.

One woman described how urinary incontinence interfered with intercourse. "I avoided sex. I was afraid I might dribble because of the pressure during intercourse." When Kegel exercises and training her bladder did not work, she opted for surgery. "It was the best decision I ever made," she says. "I am confident and turned-on again in bed. I don't worry that I am going to wet my pants when I cough or sneeze. I can even jog again."

## More Satisfying Sex
We asked about strategies for more satisfying sex that work. Here are some that were repeated often:

- Take the pressure off. Accept that your libido (and/or your partner's libido) has changed. Talk it over and laugh together. Aim for intimacy, not just sex.
- Try new things. Enjoy stroking, cuddling, hugging, and mutual masturbation. Listen to sexy music. Rent erotic videos. "We try to celebrate sexuality and intimacy in all its forms, not just intercourse," said one woman.

- Rethink your work commitments. If possible, try to synchronize your schedules. Talk with each other and learn the difference between "I'm too tired" as an excuse to avoid intimacy and "I'm too tired" when it means "I still want to be close, but I've been working eighteen hours straight."
- Get more sleep and more exercise so you don't feel so tired.
- Build in private times together. Send the kids away for the weekend. Travel; go off on a romantic holiday. Set specific times for intimate get-togethers.
- Seek help from a physician, psychologist, or a couples counselor. Try a couples workshop as a way to rejuvenate your relationship and improve communication.

Perhaps the most important advice we heard is to use your creative energy to make time for each other. When you do, intimacy will blossom. How often do you choose to stay up late to meet a deadline or prepare for the next day at work? Directing the same kind of energy at intimate sex has the potential to yield a lot more pleasure. One woman explained it this way: "We put off sex because we are both too tired. When we finally get around to doing it, we both say, 'Wow, that was good! Why don't we do this more often?'"

### Tantra for Two: Talking with the Experts

Pala Copeland and Al Link, aged fifty-two and fifty-six respectively, are the co-authors of a forthcoming book called *Soul Sex: Tantra for Two – Relationship as Spiritual Practice*. In an interview, they described Tantra: "Tantra approaches lovemaking as a way to experience exquisite union with your partner, emotionally and spiritually as well as physically. During extended Tantric lovemaking, a high sexual charge builds up which can be used for improving health, stimulating creativity, and balancing emotions."

Pala and Al offer weekend retreat workshops for couples whose ages generally range from thirty-five to fifty-five. The focus of these weekends is renewal of the couples' intimate, loving connections through disconnecting them from their everyday worlds, being taken care of, and practicing a series of Tantric exercises that Pala and Al provide. Through these exercises they encourage couples to shift away from orgasm as a goal and focus instead on deepening their emotional connection, asking each other's permission to proceed through various stages of lovemaking, and introducing the more playful, sensual pleasures of bath, massage, and sharing food.

To maintain this connection, Pala said that it is essential to allow a period of time – from two to four hours – each week to be together as lovers. Al added that setting aside this lovers' time, as difficult as it may seem to people, is "a little like saving money. You have to give to yourself first. Make a date. Write it in your calendar and keep it. That shows what your priorities really are, much more than what you say they are."

When we asked Pala and Al how they keep the spark alive in their own relationship, Al said that they start with the deliberate agreement that their relationship is the most important thing for them. They set aside a lovers' time weekly and don't let anything interfere with it. In their work with other couples, they have observed that many boomers who were part of the "free love" generation really have strong "sex-negative" messages. They seem on some level to accept that passion dies, when really it only changes. Pala and Al's approach helps couples feel hopeful. It gives them permission to be lovers again, to feel that "yes, we can do this."

To enhance lovemaking, they suggest "transforming the physical space into sacred space" by carefully tidying up and using candles, music, flowers, sensuous food, and fabric. This ritual of creating a special space can transform not only the room but the couple as well, so that they can be more present and relaxed. Pala stressed the importance of Kegel exercises, for both women and men, "every day for the rest of your life." She says the exercises will increase focus, sensitivity, and muscle tone and keep us aware of the vitality of that area of our bodies that we are so apt to ignore. For men, she says that it provides a mini prostate massage that can increase blood flow and erection capacity.

We need to remind ourselves that sexuality evolves during a lifetime, that it is different at fifty-five from what it was at twenty-five and at sixty-five from thirty-five. With the practice of lovemaking as a conscious, in-the-moment, meditative experience, a couple can share much more in both the sexual and spiritual realms.

A TANTRIC LOVING EXERCISE:
HARMONIZING YOUR BREATHING

During Tantric lovemaking, partners often harmonize their breathing and gaze deeply into each other's eyes. You can do this to achieve different effects.

- To tune into each other: At the outset of your lovers' time, sit quietly together, look into each other's eyes, and breathe in unison. This will help you tune into each other and tune out the rest of the world. Breathing slowly and deeply in this fashion will also relax you and help you focus on the present.

- To prolong sexual pleasure: When you are both highly aroused and want to prolong your pleasure by moving the energy you have built up with your love play, stop active lovemaking. For instance, if you are engaged in intercourse, stay joined but stop thrusting. Become still, look into each other's eyes, and breathe slowly and deeply together. Focus on moving your high sexual energy up from your genitals and through your whole body. This will also deepen your emotional and energetic connection.

Experiment with these variations of harmonized breathing rhythm:
- Both partners inhale and exhale at the same time.
- One partner inhales while the other exhales.

**From the Research**
*It's More Fun than a Facelift*
At Scotland's Royal Edinburgh Hospital a study of 3,500 people who looked younger than their actual ages found that having sex three times a week seemed to take seven to twelve years off their appearance. Having more sex than this did not compound the benefits, however, and casual sex seems to speed the aging process.
Source: *Health* magazine (June 2001).

*New Drugs to Treat Erectile Dysfunction*
Apomorphine – an alternative to sildenafil (Viagra) that is packaged as a
nasal spray – has been successfully tested in clinical trials and is now on the
market. It works by stimulating the hypothalamus in the brain, which in
turn stimulates erectile function. The nasal spray has few or no side-effects
and, because it works through a different mechanism than sildenafil, men
with stable angina controlled by nitrates can take it safely. It acts within
fifteen minutes of spraying, which corresponds well with the time it takes
for the onset of normal sexual response.

*New Devices to Treat Sexual Dysfunction in Women*
In 2001, Health Canada approved the Eros-Clitoris Therapy Device, the
first-ever medically approved prescription device for the treatment of
arousal disorders in women. The tiny, pliable cup is placed over the clitoris
before sex or during foreplay. Operating like the vacuum pump for men, it
moves oxygen-rich blood to the muscle in the vagina. This results in
greater lubrication and increased sensation, and it improves the woman's
ability to have an orgasm.

A female "Viagra" is also being tested, along with other creams
(alprostadil) to improve arousal and lubrication. Vitara is an over-the-
counter topical cream that is applied directly to the clitoris area before sex.
The cream makes the blood vessels dilate and makes the clitoris more sensitive. Since it is estimated that 90 per cent of female orgasms are clitoral
rather than vaginal, this drug and others like it could well increase female
sexual satisfaction and the experience of orgasm.

**On the Lighter Side**
*A Woman's Ultimate Fantasy*
Ask any man, and he will tell you that any woman's fantasy is to have two
men at once. While this has also been verified by a recent sociological study,
it appears that most men do not realize that, in this fantasy, one man is
cooking and the other man is cleaning.

*Vive la Différence*

How to Satisfy a Woman Every Time: Caress, praise, pamper, relish, savor, massage, make plans, empathize, serenade, compliment, support, feed, tantalize, bathe, humor, stroke, console, purr, hug, coddle, excite, pacify, protect, phone, correspond, anticipate, nuzzle, smooch, forgive, charm, show respect for, oblige, fascinate, attend, shower, shave, trust, defend, coax, clothe, brag about, acquiesce to, help, acknowledge, polish, spoil, embrace, accept, hear, understand, jitterbug, climb, swim, nurse, respect, entertain, calm, allay, dream about, promise, deliver, tease, flirt, commit to, enlist, pine for, murmur, snuggle with, serve, rub, rib, salve, bite, taste, nibble, gratify, swing, slip, slide, slather, mollycoddle, squeeze, moisturize, humidify, lather, tingle, keep on rockin' in the free world, wet, slicken, indulge, dazzle, amaze, flabbergast, enchant, idolize, and then start again.

How to Satisfy a Man Every Time: Show up naked.

## Questions to Reflect On

While there are no quick and easy solutions for creating a satisfying sex life, making time for intimacy, taking care of physical problems, and creating a romantic atmosphere appear to be most important. A sense of humor and lightening up also seem to be key leavening agents.

To enhance your sexual relationship, ask yourself the following questions:

1. Whether you are on your own or with a partner, what is one thing you can do for yourself to increase your sexual pleasure?
2. What is one thing you would like to tell your partner about what turns you on?
3. What is one thing you can tell your partner that you really appreciate about him or her?
4. If you are not making time for intimacy with your partner, what one step can you take to remedy that situation now?
5. Think about when you were first together. What steps can you take to re-create the atmosphere and setting that turned you on in those days?

# CHAPTER TEN

# Friends and Pets Are
# Good Medicine

Let us be grateful to people who make us happy; they are
the charming gardeners who make our souls blossom.
— Marcel Proust, *Pleasures and Regrets*, 1896

The people in our survey and our interviews – especially women – repeatedly stated that their friends are key supports in managing midlife. And as devoted dog and cat owners, we could only agree with the large number of midlife men and women who told us that their pets are good medicine.

### SOME HIGHLIGHTS FROM THE HEALTHY
### BOOMER MIDLIFE SURVEY

*Do you have at least one close friend in whom you can confide?*

|  | Men | Women |
|---|---|---|
| Yes | 85% | 97% |
| No | 15% | 3% |

*Do you belong to any community, work-related, or self-help groups?*

|  | Men | Women |
|---|---|---|
| Yes | 26% | 44% |
| No | 74% | 56% |

## On Friends

In the Healthy Boomer Midlife Survey when we asked if respondents have at least one friend they confide in, more than 90 per cent said *yes* (97 per cent of the women and 85 per cent of the men). A woman in midlife said, "My women friends have kept me going all these years. We have supported each other through a lot – having babies, building careers, coping with illness, death, teenagers, and relationship breakups. My friends have helped me stay healthy and sane through it all." One man said, "I get a lot of joy from my friends, and now that I am fifty-five years old I have the maturity to appreciate them."

There is a lot of research supporting the idea that this kind of "social support" is good for your health. Studies show that loneliness is a better predictor of mortality than high blood pressure. A person who lacks close personal ties is more prone to heart disease, cancer, depression, suicide, and emotional problems. Friendships are particularly important during an illness. People with at least one intimate confidant and several other good friends recover faster and use less medication and fewer health care services.

A recent Statistics Canada report suggests that women are particularly good at making friends. In our clinic and our interviews, this seems to hold true as well. One woman said, "I am able to talk about my deepest fears and concerns with my special women friends. Some of us have shared the years from the time our babies were born until now that they have grown up and are having their own babies. We have raged at injustices together and mourned the loss of marriages and parents. The rapport is instant. Just ten minutes' talking can make all the difference in how I feel."

A recent landmark study at UCLA (the University of California at Los Angeles) suggests that women respond to stress with a cascade of brain chemicals that cause them to make and maintain friendships with other women. This is a stunning finding that has turned five decades of stress research – most of it on men – upside down.

The researchers suspect that women have a larger behavioral repertoire than just the classic "fight or flight" response employed by men. According to Dr. Klein, a principal investigator in the UCLA study, it seems that when the hormone oxytocin is released as part of the stress response in a woman, it buffers the fight-or-flight response and encourages her to tend to children and gather with other women instead. When she engages in this "tending and befriending" behavior, more oxytocin is released in her brain, which counters stress further and produces a calming effect. This calming response does not occur in men because testosterone – which men produce in high levels when they're under stress – seems to reduce the effects of oxytocin. Women's estrogen seems to enhance it. While it may take some time to reveal all the ways that oxytocin encourages women to care for children and hang out with other women, the tend-and-befriend notion developed by Drs. Klein and Taylor may explain, at least in part, why women consistently outlive men.

Male friendships tend to differ from female ones. One man described how most of the time he spends with his best friend is spent just being with him and enjoying common interests. "There is a certain satisfaction in just sitting on the couch watching a game together or in paddling a canoe together. We don't need to be sharing intimate details about our lives to feel like we are friends." In her book *You Just Don't Understand* (1990), Deborah Tannen attributes this kind of behavior to the prehistoric days, when men moved silently in a line as they hunted animals or protected their communities. In this way they acted as a team and sacrificed for each other in times of danger or war.

"I believe that our culture and underlying fear and disapproval of homosexuality forces men to maintain a distance in same-sex relationships," one man told us. "And, at least when I was growing up, it was hard to be friends with a woman. There was always the expectation – on both sides – that friendship would lead to sex. One of the things that amazes me about the younger generation is how they make friends with the opposite sex without getting into sexual entanglements. My daughter lived in a house with another woman and a guy. She and he are still best friends and are both in committed relationships with others."

On the other hand, some men in midlife like to confide in and be friends with women because they find they can talk with them more easily. For example, in our seminars with men and in meetings with men's groups, many told us that they felt more comfortable talking with three women about personal matters that they would have felt discussing these issues with other men.

## Community Connections
In addition to having friends and acquaintances, research shows that it is good for our health to belong to at least one organization or group in the community. In the Healthy Boomer Midlife Survey, one-quarter of the men and almost half of the women who responded said they belonged

to a wide range of groups, including book and bridge clubs, women's groups, church and peace groups, professional associations, and physical activity clubs.

For almost all, belonging to these groups was positive. "I like being with other women," said one woman. "We trust each other and share common interests." Men and women who belonged to faith and spiritual groups referred to this involvement giving them comfort ("knowing that others are praying for me and my family"), satisfaction ("knowing that I am giving back to the community"), and challenge ("stimulating discussions about our life and purpose here on earth"). One woman talked about her membership in an online support group for people with STDs. "We all share a similar problem. It is anonymous and yet I feel real support and understanding coming back to me from others in the group. It is helpful."

Sports clubs and leagues – softball, tennis, basketball, ice and ball hockey, masters swim programs, and golf – were important to both sexes, and especially to men. Said one man, "I get to be with people I like, to play a game I enjoy, to feel a sense of accomplishment, to keep fit and relax all at the same time." In *Living Fit* magazine (April 1997) Toronto lawyer **Shelley Hobbs** describes how she feels to be part of a women's soccer team: "We've been a team three nights a week for six years, in rain and sleet and burning heat. I know your children. I have seen them grow up. We've car-pooled and pub-nighted and grumbled through conditioning and skill drills. I know about your brother's operation, about your Dad's Alzheimer's, about the time you wondered if your husband was having an affair. You know me, too."

For only a few, belonging to groups added to their stress. "It's just one more have-to-do," said one woman. "I quit going to the group," said another. "It made me feel frustrated and gave me a headache."

For some, membership in groups is a long-term commitment. One woman described her experience of thirty years in the same bridge club. "Some of the participants have changed over the years, but the core group has remained remarkably the same. We have grown up together." A man in his fifties describes his decision to make an Alcoholics Anonymous support group a lifetime endeavor. "They help me and I help them. We are all in it together. It helps me to continue to go."

For other boomers, joining a community group is a new experience. **Peggy** describes how she joined a book club this year – something she has always wanted to do but never made time for. "The book club is a wonderful addition to my life, partly because I get to read a good book every month. But more importantly, joining a book club has helped me make some new friends. This is not an easy thing to do when you are fifty-three and have a hectic work and family schedule. Our meetings are not very formal. We find time to ask for advice, support each other, and share personal stories over dinner, dessert, and coffee. Eventually, we get around to talking about the book . . ."

## When Friends Become Family
Sometimes friends perform important roles as family substitutes, especially for immigrants and refugees whose family members remain in the country of origin. Ottawa-based **Connie Savile** and her husband **Doug** became substitute parents for a number of young Czech immigrants who escaped to Canada when the Russian tanks rolled in in 1968. Later, they became substitute grandparents to the children of their young Czech friends. And now that "Mrs. Connie," as she is lovingly called, is eighty-eight, her midlife children stay closely in touch.

Mrs. Connie explains how the relationships began: "We read about the Czech immigrants in the paper. The community was asking for help in finding accommodation for all these new people who were arriving. My husband, Doug, asked if I was interested in taking some in. I said yes and, within a few days, we had our first couple living with us. They stayed for six months.

"I was fifty-four at the time and an 'empty nester.' My daughter was married and gone from home and our son, Harold, was working in Burlington. It was not always easy to have the young couple living in our home, but we tried to help them as much as we could. I drove them to their English classes and brought them home with a few of their friends. We all laughed as they struggled to learn English. Than I drove the others back to their homes, to save them money for the bus fares and to make sure they did not have to wait in the Ottawa cold for a bus to come."

By the time the Czech immigrants finished arriving in Ottawa, Connie and Doug knew six couples well. They were dentists, scientists, medical students, and teachers. Mrs. Connie says, "Some thirty-three years later, all of these people are still my friends. With some I am very close and we speak a few times a week; with others we call occasionally. But we never lost contact with any of them.

"When my husband was ill, they all called me and kept my spirits up. I have seen their children grow up and often drove to Toronto, Burlington, and other places to babysit if they wanted to go away. Initially, we helped them all get their homes with interest-free loans for a few years until they were able to establish their own credit and were on their feet. They all paid us back.

"Looking back, I have no regrets. It is always my Czech friends that call me now, and have done so over the years. It was a rewarding experience."

**Dr. Miroslava Lhotsky** was one of those Czech immigrants. She says, "Connie and Doug were the parents we did not have. I could go to their home when I was frustrated – either with trying to study medicine in English or to sort out difficulties in a relationship – and cry my heart out. Mrs. Connie would make hot muffins and tea, and I would go home feeling better a few hours later. Doug and Connie were always there, no matter what we were up to. Doug was always so encouraging. He believed more than I did that I could finish medical school. That was such a great gift, to know that someone honestly believes in you!

"Connie and Doug were there for our marriages and divorces, and the births of our children. They taught us how to grow a lawn; they gave us dishes to cook with. But mainly, they made us welcome in their home, any time, no matter what was going on in our lives. Connie and Doug were my Canadian family. They are grandparents to my children."

Miroslava recalls how happy Doug was to see her in the last few weeks of his life, even when his memory was failing sometimes. "I will never forget the day I visited him with Mrs. Connie. He greeted me with his honest smile and said, 'Hello darling,' as he had always done for all those thirty years. I speak to Mrs. Connie every two to three days now. We can talk about anything. She is my role model in her generosity, her acceptance of people as they are, and in her incredible vitality and joy of life. At eighty-eight, she is still full of energy and love. Doug and Mrs. Connie are my family of heart."

### Pets: Rx for Good Health

At the Baycrest Centre for Geriatric Care in North York, Ontario, Alfie, an amiable golden retriever, is a regular visitor. Patients who are lonely and dozing open their eyes, smile, pat his head, and enter into conversation as he visits each of their beds or chairs in turn.

This program and many others like it confirm what people with pets have known for years. Dogs, cats, birds, and other pets are good for your health. They provide loyal companionship, unconditional love, stimulation, routine, a sense of belonging, and good plain fun. Research documents again and again the health benefits of pets. Studies show that pet owners have fewer health problems – both minor and major. But most importantly, pets seem to have a positive effect on our mental and emotional well-being.

In the Healthy Boomer Midlife Survey, many people talked about the joy their pets brought to their daily lives. "Curling up with my cat and stroking her fur soothes away my stresses at the end of the day," said one woman. "She is also important to the children, who respect her unique personality. She is an essential part of family routines."

"My dog is my best friend and companion, especially because my husband works most evenings," said another woman. "She also gets me out walking twice a day, which ensures that I get some daily exercise. I really love the early-morning walks in the brisk air – hearing the birds and watching my neighborhood wake up."

"There is no question that walking a dog is good exercise and a good strategy for increasing your level of physical activity on a daily basis," says **Russ Kisby**, former president of ParticipACTION. One of the most popular ParticipACTION print advertisements stated:

One of the many misconceptions about exercise is that everyday activities like walking your best friend does little to improve your health. In fact, nothing could be further from the truth. The daily bound with "Spot" is great for both of you. And, considering how eager he is to go whenever you are says a lot about how little it takes to be active and feel good. Just 30 minutes a day, most days of the week, for a whole new leash . . . er, lease, on life. Of course, if you don't have a dog, there's nothing stopping you from taking yourself for a daily walk. (Leash optional.)

"This ad says it all!" declares Russ. "But walking a dog is more than just exercise. People relate to it because it is a pleasurable, everyday kind of activity. The benefits go beyond cardiovascular fitness and stronger bones. When you walk a dog you release stressful feelings. You meet people with other dogs, you stop to introduce your dog to children and you enjoy the outdoors."

One woman described the time-honored phenomenon of meeting other dog owners. "I know all the dogs' names," she says, "but few of their owners' names. It doesn't seem to matter. We talk easily about all kinds of things. Our dogs break down the barriers we commonly put up when we pass by people we don't know."

Another woman wonders if her dog has to some extent become a substitute for children in her empty nest. "I was fifty-one and all of my kids had left home when I decided to get a puppy," she explains. "Needless to say, I had forgotten that getting a puppy is a lot like bringing home an infant. She cried all night, threw up a lot, and peed on every rug in the house. One day I said to the clerk at the pet store, 'I can't believe that, after getting rid of four children, I went out and bought a puppy that needs so much care and attention.' The young salesclerk rolled her eyes and responded, 'Ma'am, you would not believe how many fifty-year-old women have told me the same thing!' "

**Strategies for Social Investing**

There is little question that investing in one's social health in midlife is every bit as important to long-term well-being as making sound financial investments. Maybe it is not just a coincidence that illness starts with "i" and wellness starts with "we." Here are some strategies for social investing that we heard from our respondents and have read about in the literature.

*Accepting Friends for Who They Are*

Both midlife men and women commented on how they were better able to forgive and indulge their friends' quirks. "I have decided that it doesn't matter if I have different political views than one of my friends," said one woman. "She and I share lots of other important things – our values about family and learning and our love of being outdoors. So I just don't bring up politics any more. I have those conversations with other friends."

One man said, "I no longer blame or criticize friends and family members the way I used to. It is time to adopt an attitude of appreciation and forgiveness. I have come to realize this as I have learned to cope with major emotional and financial challenges."

### Staying Connected with Young People

"I want to be just like my mother-in-law," said one woman. "At age eighty-one she is vibrant and interested in life. She still runs a business in the summer and is an active volunteer. I believe that one of her secrets is having friends of all ages. She socializes and works with younger adults who look to her for advice. Every week in the summer she hosts a party for the children who are camping at her lodge. She has as good a time as they do, playing games, singing camp songs, and roasting marshmallows."

A midlife man who does not have children of his own says that "volunteering with troubled kids sometimes makes me realize how old I am, but mostly it keeps me feeling young, involved, and happy that I can be of some help."

A midlife couple that runs their own business describe how mentoring young people is important to them. "It helps us stay current and it keeps the business vibrant. It is part of our succession planning. But most importantly, interacting with younger people is fun. Our days and our lives are richer for it."

### Nurturing All Types of Friends

In her book *Necessary Losses* (1986), Judith Viorst describes four types of friends:

- *Convenience friends* are those whose lives routinely intersect with ours (for example, neighbors and car-pool partners). We are close but not too close. They provide us with stability and regular social contact and will help out in a pinch.
- *Special-interest friends* do things with us, such as play tennis at the club or collect for the Cancer Society. In the *Medical Post*

(October 16, 2001), Dr. Robert Weil, a ninety-two-year-old psychiatrist, writes, "Western culture has an implacable aversion to aging. I want to offer some personal advice to those who, like me, are trying to avoid despair or disgust, and discover the virtues of aging. Friendships are by far the best part of aging. For years I would meet regularly with a group of people at a restaurant. As you age, there is a certain continuity or comfort level you reach when you spend time with people who share common interests."

- *Historical or crossroads friends* are those we grew up with. They knew us way back when we were little or shared a special time with us, such as studying at university. One woman described how she feels whenever she reconnects with her old college roommate: "It is like we have never been apart, even though we only see each other once or twice a year. We have gone our separate ways in different cities, but the special intimacy is still there. We just pick up where we left off."

- *Friends of the heart* (Viorst calls them "generational friends") – are those special, intimate friends to whom you can tell anything, even things you might not be able to discuss with an intimate partner. They are the ones who you can call at 2:00 in the morning, and they will always respond. Friends of the heart transcend time and space. These are the ones you hold on to.

Midlife is a time for recognizing, cultivating, and enjoying all of these types of friends. Friends give us pleasure and contribute to our personal growth. But most important are the close friends to whom we can turn for reassurance and guidance as we traverse midlife. "My best friend told me I am okay, even when I acted like an idiot when I went through my divorce," said one woman. "At the time I really needed her to stand by me. She didn't criticize me like everyone else did. She said that I was still me, and still her best friend, and that I was going through a hard time and a big loss. She said that I was okay!"

A number of people told us about their efforts to reconnect with historical friends, especially high-school buddies. One woman found an old friend on a high-school website. They reconnected by e-mail, then arranged to meet. Now they keep in touch on a regular basis. Another man described how an old high-school football buddy called and suggested that five old friends take a ski holiday. "We skied our buns off and reminisced. It turned out that two of them were members of AA so we all went to their support meeting. I guess we came full circle – going from drinking buddies to recovery buddies." Now the ski trip is an annual event.

Several people talked about that unique event called the twenty-five-year class reunion. "I was terrified," admitted one woman, "that my old inadequacies would resurface. I felt more confidence when a lot of other people – including the hotshots from my day – said they felt the same way. I was struck with the fact that the women looked pretty well the same as I remembered. But we kept saying to each other, 'What happened to the men? How come they are all bald and have big stomachs?'" Several people talked about the shock of finding that some of their old colleagues were dead, mostly from cancer. At least one couple reestablished a high-school romance at their reunion and is now happily married.

### From the Research
*Staying Connected Is as Important as Not Smoking*
Research on social support and social isolation shows that death rates for socially isolated adults are two to three times higher than rates for socially integrated adults. Public-health experts have concluded that the association between your support networks and your health is now as strong as the epidemiological evidence linking smoking and health.
Source: Gironda, M., and J. Lubben, "Preventing Loneliness and Isolation in Older Adulthood." In Gullotta, T., and M. Bloom (eds.). *Encyclopedia of Primary Prevention and Health Promotion*. New York: Kluwer Academic/Plenum Publishers (forthcoming, 2002).

### Understanding Loneliness
Loneliness is the feeling of being emotionally apart from others. As people grow older, their social networks may shrink, because they have outlived relatives and friends, suffer from chronic health problems that limit their mobility, and experience limited social opportunities, which results in social isolation. This type of loneliness is remedied by increasing involvement with family, peers, friends, and neighbors. Affectionate relationships

with children and a perceived availability of family and peer contacts are key buffers against loneliness for older people.

Source: Gironda, M., and J. Lubben, "Preventing Loneliness and Isolation in Older Adulthood." In Gullotta, T., and M. Bloom (eds.). *Encyclopedia of Primary Prevention and Health Promotion*. New York: Kluwer Academic/Plenum Publishers (forthcoming, 2002).

## On the Lighter Side
*The Senility Friendship Prayer*
God, grant me the senility to forget the people I never liked anyway, the good fortune to run into the ones that I do, and the eyesight to tell the difference.

*Lessons from a Dog*
1. When loved ones come home, always run to greet them.
2. Take naps and always stretch before rising.
3. Run, romp, and play daily.
4. Eat with gusto and enthusiasm.
5. Be loyal.
6. If what you want lies buried, dig until you find it.
7. When someone is having a bad day, be silent, sit close by, and nuzzle them gently.
8. Delight in the simple joy of a long walk.
9. Thrive on attention and let people touch you.
10. Avoid biting when a simple growl will do.
11. When you are happy, dance around and wag your entire body.
12. No matter how often you are criticized, don't buy into the guilt thing and pout. Run right back and make friends.

## Questions to Reflect On
In midlife, we become more conscious of how important relationships with friends and animals really are to us. With some strategic social investing we can ensure that our years to come will be filled with the comfort and joy that positive personal connections can bring.

1. What is one step you can take now to acknowledge and strengthen your relationships with your intimate friends of the heart?

2. Which old (historical) friends would you like to reconnect with? How will you do this in the next six months?

3. Do you have friends of all ages? If not, how can you cultivate one friend who is younger than you and one friend who is older than you?

4. Do you participate in a community organization, group, or club? If no, is there one you would like to join? What can you do now to find out more about joining this group?

5. If you have a pet, what small thing can you do to increase the time and enjoyment you have with your pet?

6. If you do not have a pet and would like to get one, ask yourself if you are currently in a position to provide a good home. If the answer is yes, talk to the people you live with about the possibility of getting a pet.

# CHAPTER ELEVEN

# *An Attitude of Gratitude*

Gratitude unlocks the fullness of life. It turns what we have into enough, and more. It turns denial into acceptance, chaos to order, confusion to clarity. It can turn a meal into a feast, a house into a home, a stranger into a friend. Gratitude makes sense of our past, brings peace for today, and creates a vision for tomorrow.

– Melody Beattie, *Codependent No More*, 1987

Historians may categorize North American boomers as "the spoiled generation." Our group is large and influential. We have grown up in a period with no world wars, relative economic prosperity, massive technological advances, and improved access to higher education. Many of us were indulged by parents determined to give us more than they had. We are the recipients of hard-won rights for sex and racial equality and are the first generation to experience the sexual freedom of adequate birth-control methods. After all, isn't it the boomers' birthright to have the best music, the best cars, perfect families, and satisfying careers?

So why does happiness evade so many boomers? Why do we often catch ourselves complaining, "Someone just cut me off with his car; the kitchen renovations that were to be finished weeks ago are lingering on; no one appreciates me at work . . ."

Maybe it is time to stop for a moment – to count our blessings and cultivate what has been dubbed "an attitude of gratitude." This idea was raised repeatedly by those who answered the questions in the Healthy Boomer Midlife Survey. One fifty-five-year-old woman said, "I try to remember that life is short, that no one I know has died wishing to spend more time at the office, that I have been granted the great good fortune to have a standard of living that is better than that of 99 per cent of people on this planet.

It is rude to reject or ignore such a gift. When I keep this in my mind on a daily basis, my gratitude gives me balance as well as happiness."

### Cultivating an Attitude of Gratitude

John Fitzgerald Kennedy, the assassinated American president and a hero for many boomers, once said, "As we express our gratitude, we must never forget that the highest appreciation is not to utter words, but to live by them." Easier said than done. How does one cultivate an attitude of gratitude and then live by this philosophy? The respondents to our survey, combined with a host of popular books on today's shelves, suggest some helpful strategies.

*Focusing on the Positive*

One boomer described her father, Ted, who is eighty-six years old and has severe arthritis that limits his mobility and causes him a lot of pain. Yet he never complains. He finds something positive in everything that happens each day. He remains enthusiastic about every outing, every visit, even the sighting of a bird in his backyard.

Why do people like Ted remain joyful in difficult situations while others lead what Henry David Thoreau called "lives of quiet desperation"? "It's all in your attitude," says Ted. "I learned early on that complaining is catching. Life is too precious to waste it being negative and unhappy."

Sometimes life throws us some very challenging curves. When this happens, we need to work to recast a situation in a positive light. This is precisely what one of our respondents did when she was diagnosed with cancer in her mid-fifties.

"For the first few days after I was confronted with a cancer diagnosis, I felt angry and sorry for myself. Than it dawned on me, that I am actually very lucky! At age twenty-seven, I had been involved in a very serious car accident. It was a miracle that I lived and completely regained my health. Suddenly, I realized how much has happened in the thirty years since the accident. I met my husband, had my children, and have enjoyed such a full life up till now. I could have missed all of this. Suddenly, this new ordeal I was facing became bearable. I felt energized knowing that it is how we live, not just the time we 'put in' that counts."

Most of us are devastated by the loss of a job. But, **Alan**, a fifty-three-year-old executive who has experienced company downsizing several times in his career has learned to interpret the dreaded announcement of company restructuring positively.

He says, "When I see a plan to restructure coming up, I get ready. In fact, I am facing a downsizing of my company right now. Fifty-four people may have to go. I may be of them, I may not; but I am getting ready nonetheless. I used to work in advertising, so I have learned to be adaptive and creative about handling change. Rather than brooding and worrying, I look at it as a challenge to create a new job for myself. This makes me feel excited and challenged. And I have a more interesting life by being adaptable . . ."

"I was raised in a family of pessimists," said another man. "Now I try to catch myself when I have a negative reaction to an everyday occurrence. I think about a positive result instead of predicting a negative. This makes a big difference in how people react to me and how stressed I feel at the end of the day."

*Focusing on What You Have, Not on What You Don't Have*
In many of our interviews, people spoke about the need to focus on what we have, rather than on what we do not have. **Flora MacDonald**, former Canadian cabinet minister, has spent the last twelve years working in developing countries on issues such as aging, health, development, and human rights. (See Chapter 7 for more of her interview.)

She says, "It discourages me to hear Canadians complain about what they don't have when I look at how people in developing countries cope with such difficult conditions. We have so much to be grateful for in Canada. And we have a lot to learn from the perseverance, courage, and sense of humor people in developing countries display in the face of almost overwhelming barriers."

Reflecting on our good fortunes means consciously reminding ourselves of what we have. One of our respondents said, "When I was younger, I took everything for granted. I had little understanding of the importance of humility. Now, I take nothing for granted. I feel very grateful for all the richness in my life." Another woman, aged fifty-two, said, "I try to feel grateful rather than guilty for all that I have."

Oprah Winfrey and Sarah Ban Breathnach, author of the popular book *Simple Abundance* (1995), have a practical suggestion for how we can account for what we have. They both keep a Gratitude Journal, in which, at the end of each day, they record five simple things for which they are grateful.

### Cherishing Your Family and Friends

Relationships with partners, family members – especially children and grandchildren – and friends were cited repeatedly as a key reason why we should be grateful in midlife. Here is a typical response from a fifty-five-year-old woman: "What gives me joy in midlife? Relationships with friends, parents, and siblings, my four amazing, wonderful children, my grandchildren. And, sometimes, feeling wise." Another woman said, "I find most pleasure in loving relationships – a caring, loving man who feels the same about me; good, solid relationships with friends; meaningful conversations." One fifty-five-year-old man said, "There are many little joys, but being loved for who I am is the most joyous of all." The importance of relationships to well-being in midlife is explored further in Chapters 8 and 12.

### Appreciating the Simple Pleasures of Everyday Life

September 11, 2001, provided further impetus for boomers to reevaluate their personal attitudes toward life and to be more grateful for the freedom and pleasures of each day that we can so easily take for granted. But do we need to be shaken by a calamity, global or personal, to appreciate the small things in our lives?

In our survey, the simple pleasures of everyday life ranked second after relationships with family members and friends in midlife. Other such pleasures included:

- taking a few minutes each day to appreciate nature, to go for a walk and notice the beautiful leaves;
- home life and spending time with my partner;
- being engaged in daily life;
- my dogs, flowers, and gardening;
- speaking my mind, laughter;
- beauty, kindness, stillness;

- music, reading;
- seeking new experiences through travel.

## Living in the Moment

Spiritual leaders such as the Dalai Lama and the Vietnamese Buddhist monk Thich Nhat Hanh link cultivating a gratitude for life with the experience of being in the present, right here, right now. Thich Nhat Hanh calls this the practice of mindfulness. He suggests having mantras (short repetitive prayers) for simple daily events, such as expressing an internal thank you for the miracle of water each time we turn on the faucet or using a red light while driving as an opportunity to take three deep breaths. In this way, one replaces one's inner mindless chatter with moments of grateful awareness. As one woman said, "When our family says grace before a meal, it gives us all a chance to be quiet inside. It allows us to let go of the busyness of the day and appreciate each other and what we are about to eat."

## Practicing "Random Acts of Kindness"

The movement for "random acts of kindness" became popular in the United States in the early 1990s as an effort to counterbalance the "random acts of senseless violence" that have become far too frequent in modern society.

Perpetrators of guerilla goodness always leave an item in the food-bank bin when they buy groceries. They anonymously bring flowers to the office, smile as they let in a driver merging onto a busy road, and compliment a bus driver on his competent service. They send thank-you e-mails to colleagues on the completion of a project, anonymously leave a new basketball at the local Boys and Girls Club, stop to help stranded drivers, or pay the entrance fee to the local swimming pool for the two children behind them when they pay their own.

Why do they do it? One boomer explains her philosophy: "I read about it and thought it was a neat, fun idea. I started to buy eight jars of baby food every time I went shopping, and left them in the food-bank bin. I had heard on the radio that the food banks always need baby food. After I had done it a few times, it became more than a fun idea. It was an efficient, easy way for me to give something anonymously every time I filled my cart and realized how well my family can afford to eat. I imagine the stressed young moms who are happy to get baby food for their little ones, and I feel good. It's only a little thing, but it has become important to me. I like myself better for doing it."

Giving a gift of kindness, big or small, to someone you know or don't know, is an old idea that we badly need as a society in modern times. Boomers who practice it quickly discover that it feels good and that people are kinder to them in return.

*Learning to Value the Wisdom That Comes with Age and Experience*
Men and women in midlife are unhappy about the indignities of aging: sagging skin, protruding tummies, graying hair, and memory lapses. But it was heartening to see in our survey that some boomers are also learning to value and enjoy the wisdom and experience they have gained along the way. "It gets easier when you listen to the wisdom you've been building up over the years," said one woman. "It's time we gave ourselves some credit for what we have learned and for our years of striving to be a better person."

In the 1960s, Theodore Roszak, a history professor at California State University, began documenting the development of the youthful revolution of consciousness. After three decades and a nearly fatal bout with heart disease, he examined the emergence of another major cultural development in *America the Wise: The Longevity Revolution and the True Wealth of Nations* (New York: Houghton Mifflin, 1998).

In this book, he describes wisdom this way:

> Wisdom is examined experience, examined in the same way Socrates examined all that his pupils said, helping them find their way through their thoughts, offering a word of criticism here, a word of encouragement there, bringing them to view the values and presuppositions that underlay their beliefs with discriminating distance. Wisdom grows from any ordinary life, provided that life is taken seriously and brought under reflection. That is all wisdom is, yet it is infinitely precious and wholly indispensable to growing up.

As members of the Big Generation become the elders of modern society, we need to recognize and be grateful that wisdom is a gift we can all gain through simple reflection. It is not the exclusive territory of academics, specialists, and technocrats.

We asked, "Now that you are in midlife, what gives you the most joy in life?" Here are the top six answers:

1. Loving relationships: spending time with my partner and other family members.
2. Being part of the growth and development of my children and grandchildren.
3. Interacting and laughing with friends and pets.
4. Enjoying the simple things in life: reading in bed in a flannel nightie, going to the beach, watching the sun go down, enjoying martinis, taking time to enjoy sewing, meditating, travel, adventures.
5. Mastery and growth: using my talents, getting things done, accomplishing things at work, learning new things.
6. Helping others, volunteering, making a difference in others' lives.

## Helping You Helps Me

Many boomers are searching for ways to give something back to their communities by volunteering their personal time and skills. In the process, they find that many benefits come back to them. One fifty-six-year-old woman said, "I volunteer as a Reading Buddy once a week at a local public school. It gives me something to think about and plan for. Volunteering makes me feel good. I am giving something back to society."

A fifty-year-old man described both his formal and informal contributions: "I sit on the board of an international development organization. I also organize an annual neighborhood golf tournament. I enjoy my volunteer activities very much. They give me a sense of contribution and achievement."

Another man in his late fifties referred to the new skills he had learned through volunteer work. "I took on a voluntary leadership role after I retired in an area where I had little experience. This necessitated new challenges and new learning. It was a stimulating, interesting, and rewarding experience."

Canadian historian **Ramsay Cook** took on some volunteer work in his retirement that was unrelated to his esteemed career as a Canadian historian. He worked as a volunteer in Toronto's Daily Food Bank half a day a week. "It was a great experience," says Ramsay. "My most striking finding was that the people who came to the food bank were not drunks or people who did not want to work, as most people presume, but an average kind of people who for various reasons were struggling at this time to get food on the table. It was great to see how volunteer organizations work and how many people – especially older people – are actively volunteering." (For more on how Cook deals with retirement, see notes from his interview in Chapter 7, "Will My Money Run Out Before I Do?")

According to the 2000 Canadian National Survey of Giving, Volunteering and Participating, 76 per cent of volunteers reported gaining interpersonal skills, such as understanding people better, motivating others, and dealing with difficult situations. Sixty-six per cent said they developed communication skills in public speaking, writing, conducting meetings, and public relations. Sixty-four per cent reported gaining knowledge about such issues as health, women's concerns, politics, criminal justice, and the environment.

When **Larry** retired from his post in the dean's office at a university school of mathematics, he decided to volunteer with a local support service group that provides transportation and shopping help to older people who are no longer mobile enough to do it themselves. "I had been shopping for my mother for a number of years. I knew the stores or and thought that it made sense to do it for some others as well."

He is now in his sixth year as a volunteer shopper. He has anywhere from three to five "clients" at a time, all of whom are in their eighties. He spends every Friday on his shopping work. He goes to each house, picks up a list, and confirms the various brands and types of food that his clients want. "Most have not been a store for a while, and they are unaware of the wide variety of choices now. I will go to different stores to get their preferences, but I also tell them when I know there is a better deal on a particular brand or in a particular store." He gets the items they need, brings them back, settles the accounts with them, and spends some time talking with each of the women. "I try to work in time for a visit," he says, "especially for those who are lonely and have no relatives in the city."

Larry goes the extra mile for his clients. In addition to the shopping, he takes them out in his car to see the Christmas lights in December, and he and his wife invite all the women to dinner at their house. "They get to know each other pretty quickly and find they have common friends and interests when we do our get-togethers," says Larry.

Larry is the only male volunteer in his local service group who takes on the shopping assignments. "I try to convince other men to do it, to but they say that grocery shopping is not their thing. However, some have volunteered to drive older people to appointments." What does he get out of his unique volunteer work? "I have lived in this community all of my life," he says, "and it is a small way of giving back. These seniors don't want to be a burden. It feels good to be able to help them remain independent in their own homes. I get joy out of their joy and their sincere thank-yous really cheer me up."

**Mary Jane** received the President's Award from the United Way in recognition of her outstanding work with that organization: "I felt a little embarrassed; it certainly wasn't expected. I got involved as a result of a suggestion from a friend. I helped them out with strategic planning and training – activities that fit with my skill set and professional work. I didn't think of it as a big deal, although I did recognize that it was a major time commitment. As usual when you give, I got more back than I gave. It enriched my life. I met some wonderful people and I felt good about making a contribution."

She has another motivation for volunteering – to serve as a role model for her three children and grandchildren. "Having an outer view and contributing to the community are a life value for me that I learned from my parents. I wanted to pass this on to my own children. When they were young, I was involved in activities with them. I coached soccer and they helped me at volunteer bazaars. As they got older, they did their own volunteer activities, and I took on different kinds of things.

"My father was the 'master of the magnanimous gesture.' He used to give spontaneously to anyone who needed it. I remember one day as a child watching him quietly give a man money in a line at a department store, because he could not get credit for a purchase he really needed. My father's philosophy was simple: give without conditions and leave the dignity of the person you give to intact."

Her parents' spirit and habit of giving has had a powerful influence on all seven of their children, their grandchildren, and their great-grandchildren. At Christmas they all participate in buying, wrapping, and taking gifts to the Shepherds of Good Hope, instead of buying presents for each other. "We make it a family ritual that is fun to do. Wrapping the gifts together and taking them as a group makes it a lot more meaningful than just giving money."

Last year, when her sister heard that a young struggling family had lost most of their possessions in a robbery, Mary Jane got her family organized. Together, they rounded up household furnishings, a television, a VCR, and other items. They added some new bedding and helped with the rent for a few months. Three months later, another family member heard on his car radio that there had been a fire in a downtown apartment. He recognized the address and drove to the scene, where he found the same family totally burned out. The response from Mary Jane's family was predictable. They quietly and efficiently refurnished the apartment again.

Studies have noted a number of measurable health benefits associated with volunteering and giving, including lowered blood pressure, improved immune-system function, and enhanced self-esteem. One Cornell University study found that, among 762 retired people, those who volunteered were happier than non-volunteers and had more energy and a greater sense of control over their lives. According to the boomers in our survey, taking the time to find and contribute to volunteer activities enhances your well-being.

Boomers have many choices about volunteering. Many people use the experience and the contacts they have built up over the years. Others try something entirely new. Some prefer to work with religious groups or established organizations for causes that have affected family members, such as the Cancer Society or the Diabetes Association. Mary Jane suggests that people keep their ears open and use existing networks to find volunteer activities that appeal to them. "Most people are more comfortable when they can use existing skill sets," she suggests. "It is also important to give to a cause or issue that has personal meaning. For example, my brother had an important personal experience with the children's hospital, so it is natural for him and his family to help them out. Lastly, every city and town has a volunteer bureau. People can always contact them for ideas."

When asked how she finds the time for volunteer work in her busy schedule, Mary Jane laughs. "You know the old saying, give a busy person the job. It's true. I have learned to be organized and to build my voluntary time into my schedule. People should not fool themselves. You can choose to give as much time as you want, but working with volunteer agencies is a commitment, just like paid work. Sometimes your employer gives you 'time off' to go to meetings, but this is a false economy. Your office work is still there when you get back, so you end up taking it home or staying late."

Some successfully establish their own voluntary organizations. This is what Murray Dryden from Islington, Ontario, did. In 1970 at age fifty-eight, he launched Sleeping Children Around the World (SCAW) with his wife, Margaret. SCAW provides bed kits, each consisting of a frame and slats, mattress, sheet, woolen blanket, pillow and case, and pajamas, for children all over the world. For more than twenty-five years, SCAW has provided some 350,000 bed kits for children in twenty-nine countries. Thirty volunteers run the organization out of the Dryden home, which has neither administrative overheads nor government funding.

**From the Research**
*Patterns of Volunteering*
Thirty-seven per cent of Canadians thirty-five to forty-four years old volunteer, making them more likely to contribute than any other age group. Rates of volunteering tend to remain high until age sixty-five when they start to decline. However, seniors contribute the greatest amount of time annually – 202 hours on average. Women are more likely to volunteer than men are, although when men volunteer they tend to contribute more hours annually than women do. Here are some key reasons why boomers volunteer:

- involvement in children's educational and recreational activities;
- to help a cause in which they personally believe;

- because they have been personally affected or know someone who has been personally affected by the cause the organization supports.

Source: Government of Canada. *Caring Canadians, Involved Canadians: Highlights from the 1997 National Survey of Giving, Volunteering and Participating.* Ottawa: Department of Industry, 1998.

## On the Lighter Side

*Are You an Optimist or a Pessimist?*

Optimistic people are more likely than negative thinkers to assume an attitude of gratitude. Research has also shown that optimists live longer, healthier lives than pessimists do. If you are an optimist, you believe that bad events such a car accident have temporary, specific causes such as a sudden downpour or bad headlights. You also believe that good things can always be found in any situation. Pessimists, of course, believe just the opposite. Here is a story about two twins – one an optimist and the other a pessimist.

A family had twin boys whose only resemblance to each other was their looks. One was an eternal optimist, the other a doom-and-gloom pessimist. Just to see what would happen, on Christmas night their father loaded the pessimist's room with every imaginable toy and game. He loaded the optimist's room with horse manure.

Later, he found the pessimist sitting amid his new gifts crying bitterly.

"Why are you crying?" the father asked.

"Because my friends will be jealous. I'll have to read all these instructions before I can do anything with this stuff. I'll constantly need batteries, and my toys will eventually get broken," answered the pessimistic twin.

Passing the optimist twin's room, the father found him dancing for joy in the pile of manure. "What are you so happy about?" he asked.

To which his optimist son replied, "Somewhere in here, there has got to be a pony!"

## Questions to Reflect On

When we asked people what gives them joy in midlife, their answers referred to relating, sharing, giving, mastery, and simple pleasures – all vital ingredients in nurturing an attitude of gratefulness in our lives. When we feel grateful, we are much less likely to feel hard done by, resentful, and irritated. We are better able to see the big picture, keep things in perspective, and not sweat the small stuff. A daily practice of gratitude can contribute greatly to keeping us physically and emotionally healthy.

1. What makes you feel grateful to be alive today? Write down three specific things.
2. How can you reframe a negative attitude toward a troubling situation you are currently experiencing as more positive?
3. What random act of kindness will you do today?
4. If you are not already a volunteer, would you consider voluntarily contributing your time and skills? What kind of volunteer work would interest you? What small step can you take to prepare for this or to start now?

# CHAPTER TWELVE

# The End of Summer:
# Healthy Boomers Never Die . . .
# or Even Get Old, Do They?

When death comes
like the hungry bear in autumn;
when death comes and takes all the bright coins from his purse

to buy me, and snaps the purse shut;
. . . . . . . . . . . . . . . . . . . . . . . . .
When it's over, I want to say: all my life
I was a bride married to amazement.
I was the bridegroom, taking the world into my arms.

When it's over, I don't want to wonder
if I have made of my life something particular and real.
I don't want to find myself sighing and frightened,
or full of argument.

I don't want to end up simply having visited this world.
– Mary Oliver, "When Death Comes,"<br>
*New and Selected Poems,* 1992

For many boomers, the poignant truth of Mary Oliver's words begins to assume new meaning in midlife. We may not think of ourselves as being in the autumn of our lives yet, but we know that spring has passed and we are closer to the end of the summer than the beginning. Our eyes, our joints, and our mirrors tell us that we are getting older. Sometimes we feel despondent or frightened or full of denial about the middle passage in which we find ourselves. As parents and friends become sick and die, or as we ourselves are challenged by life-threatening illnesses, we can no longer continue to resist the reality of death, as we have tried so hard to do in the past.

For most North American boomers, dying has been removed from our homes and our daily lives. As we grew up, we went to funerals in the impersonal surroundings of "the funeral home." We saw dead people looking as if they were not old or emaciated from the illness that took them, but rather propped up and in full makeup, looking ready for Madame Tussaud's museum.

When we asked people about their experiences of aging, death, and dying, their answers were rich and complex. In this chapter, we present their reflections in the hope that they will help us deal with our own reluctance to embrace aging and our fears about dying. Most importantly, we hope that sharing what we have learned will help all of us to live more fully in the moments we have right now.

## Confronting Aging

Imagine you are in a spaceship fifty years from now looking down on earth. You see attractive, productive earthlings of all ages. But you wonder about the strange group you see jogging three times a day in their gated communities, shut off from the rest of society. They are more than a hundred years of age and *very* thin – after all, one of the latest theories on the planet is that extreme calorie reduction is one way to live longer. They survive mostly on vegetable juices and supplements. Most of their joints and bones are plastic; years of starvation and running on pavement have taken a toll. They are wearing the latest brand of jogging shoes and sports clothes. A permanent, synthetic covering over their skin protects them from the sun and gives them a perpetual, youthful-looking tan. Their faces are smooth and their buttocks are tight, but the skin on their chests and arms gives away their age. They all have flowing locks of hair; however, when you look closely you can see the roots of the transplanted hair follicles. These earthlings are smiling and pretending to have fun, but beneath the levity you can see they are lonely and afraid. You wonder why they cannot let themselves age gracefully and die with dignity. Maybe they are an anti-aging experiment their so-called boomer generation was forced to carry out for the good of their species . . .

Sound preposterous? Sometimes we wonder. According to the

Internet and almost daily headlines, our generation stands at the fore-front of scientific discoveries and "magic" regimens that could stop or reverse the whole aging process. Boomers spend millions of dollars on anti-aging potions, hormones, supplements, fad diets, creams, cleansers, and surgical operations. We read eagerly about experimental treatments with melatonin, antioxidants, growth hormones, and other regimens designed to "cure" aging and create the illusion that we may just be able to beat our mortality.

One wonders if our generation's inability to confront aging and ulti-mately death, combined with our unwavering faith in science, is driving an agenda that employs cloning, embryonic stem cells, and genetic alterations in a great attempt to eliminate dying completely.

At the same time that the Big Generation continues to fight against growing older, we face a paradox. Worldwide aging is not a negative phe-nomenon. It is in fact one of the greatest triumphs of our time. North Americans can now expect to live to age eighty, compared to only fifty years a century ago. The proportion of "old-old" people – more than eighty years of age – is growing faster than any other age group. The number of cente-narians in England has grown so quickly that the Queen no longer sends a congratulatory note to each British citizen who turns a hundred. There are some seventy-two thousand people older than a hundred years living in the American New England states alone – and it is now believed that many of them originally came from Nova Scotia. Most industrial countries boast about one centenarian for every ten thousand people. In Nova Scotia, there are two per ten thousand! This means that this Canadian maritime province boasts a higher proportion of centenarians than anywhere in North America, possibly the planet!

All of us know some eighty-five- or ninety-year-old men and women who are still active in culture, the arts, learning, and family and community life. Some of them help take care of "younger" friends in their seventies. All of them find something to be joyful about in their daily lives. These women and men are not fighting against aging. On the contrary, they are proud of their longevity. One woman talked about her ninety-eight-year-old father, who still walks and plays the piano every day. "Papa seems to get a certain pleasure out of reading the obituaries – because his name is not there! He is beating the odds, getting a few more days or weeks or months or years.

It's not because he is greedy. He is proud to have lived this long. He just finds joy in being alive."

Boomers can learn a lot from these older role models. There is little point in fearing the aging process and denying the death that will inevitably follow. Why not celebrate our health and the accomplishments of aging instead?

### Forging New Images of Aging

Boomers are not only living longer; we are living better. Several years ago, trends forecaster Faith Popcorn identified a phenomenon she called "down-aging." She was referring to how most people now experience at age seventy-five the kind of physical declines that our grandparents experienced at age sixty-five. In other words, we have gained ten years in terms of health and quality of life in just two generations.

More than any other group, the boomers have altered and continue to alter our perceptions of youth, middle age, and old age. As a result, there have also been dramatic changes in the social norms that have traditionally accompanied those transitions. Two hundred years ago, Jane Austen acknowledged that, at age thirty, youth was behind her and she was no longer eligible for marriage. Today, most young adults are delaying marriage until their mid-twenties or later, if they decide to marry at all. Midlife adults are marrying for the first time, remarrying and creating second families, cohabiting, or choosing to live apart while maintaining committed relationships. Some are taking on the parenting role in their mid- to late forties. Boomers are embarking on new careers and running marathons in their fifties. They are flooding community colleges and inventing new ways to go back to school through online courses and virtual learning centers.

The chronological period commonly referred to as "midlife" has expanded to encompass ages forty to sixty-five. But increasingly, boomers are asking if chronological age matters at all. As Doris Lessing writes in *The Summer Before the Dark* (1973), "You are young and then you are middle-aged, but it is hard to tell the moment of passage from one state to the next." The Big Generation balks at such labels as "senior citizen" that are linked to age, even though some of us are happy to cash in on travel and hotel discounts that are increasingly offered to "seniors" at age fifty-five!

Historically, midlife menopause has been associated with the end of youth, sexuality, beauty, and reproductive usefulness. In an 1871 publication entitled *Physical Life of a Woman: Advice to the Maiden, Wife and Mother*, author G. H. Naphey describes the menopausal woman as "depressed, fretful, peevish, annoying to all those around her and impossible to live with." He believed that her sufferings were part of Mother Nature's plan "to deprive her forever of taking part in the creative act after a certain age." Even today, menopause is often seen as a "deficiency," a disease that represents the end of sexual attractiveness and needs to be corrected with hormone replacement therapy.

As boomer women start to move into menopause in large numbers, attitudes toward this time of life are changing dramatically. The silence has been broken with a plethora of books, videos, talk shows, support groups, and jokes about hot flashes, mammograms, mood swings, and other symptoms associated with the perimenopause and menopause. Happily, most stereotypes and myths from the past have largely been negated and forgotten. Many North American women feel freer after menopause because they no longer have to worry about pregnancy or about competing for the men that Mother Nature wants them to reproduce with.

The boomers are also exploring new attitudes toward men's experience of aging in midlife, drawing important parallels between the male experience and the menopause experience for women. Forty per cent of the men who responded to the Healthy Boomer Midlife Survey said that they believed that a male menopause (andropause) exists; 18 per cent stated that it did not exist and 42 per cent said that they did not know whether or not it exists. Many men talked about the same complaints that women had identified, especially weight gain, fatigue, and an increase in fat around the abdomen. The men were more likely than women to be troubled by a loss of muscle mass, decreased endurance, poorer overall fitness, and performances in sports. "I tire a lot sooner when I am physically active," said one man. "I don't know if this is male menopause or just aging, but I sure don't like it much."

## Our Denial of Death

Our youth-oriented culture that so avoids aging and death has moved us away more and more from the reality of death. Death is something we watch from a safe distance on television or at the movies. For most of us, death is neither a familiar nor a comfortable part of our lives.

In his article "Death's Gift to Life" in *Maclean's* magazine (December 17, 2001), journalist Ron Graham writes,

> Modern American culture, shaped as it's been by extended periods of prosperity and peace, has been remarkably successful in suppressing the reality of death. We banish our chronically ill to institutions. We lock ourselves behind alarm systems and gated communities. We dream up Star Wars shields to protect our continent from foreign missiles. Naively safe, we dwell in a fool's paradise of eternal youth.

Because of the extraordinary technological advances in medicine during our lifetime, we now face ethical dilemmas about illness and death that were undreamed of in previous generations. Should we keep loved ones on life-prolonging machinery when their deaths are imminent? Would we want this for ourselves? Does an older person with a serious health problem really benefit from invasive procedures that may compromise his or her quality of life in the long run? In other words, is longer life at any cost always the best choice? Should those who suffer many other illnesses associated with aging have these aggressive interventions? Should those who are in pain and wish to die be assisted if they request it?

These are no longer academic questions for boomers who are dealing with their parents' illnesses and deaths and beginning to face their own mortality. After years of avoidance and denial of the subject, most of us are woefully unprepared to make calm and thoughtful choices when the times of decision suddenly arrive.

### SOME HIGHLIGHTS FROM THE HEALTHY BOOMER MIDLIFE SURVEY

*If you could choose, at what age would you choose to die?*

| Age | Percentage |
| --- | --- |
| 99 years and older | 22% |
| 90–98 years | 20% |
| 80–89 years | 38% |
| No answer | 20% |

---

*What is your biggest worry about getting older and dying?*
1. Dying alone and in pain.
2. Losing who I am; becoming completely dependent on others.
3. Being poor and sick.
4. Leaving young children behind if death comes too soon; leaving my family with unresolved problems.
5. Losing my partner and close friends.
6. Being cared for in a large institution with no friends or family nearby.
7. Having a prolonged and agonizing death; being kept on life support.
8. The finality of death.

---

When we asked our survey respondents how long they want to live, most said they'd like to live to age ninety or older. One woman quipped, "I plan to die at age one hundred, shot dead on the dance floor by a jealous lover. Seriously though, I hope to die peacefully when my time comes, with no pain."

As a generation that has experienced an unprecedented degree of control over birth control, fertility, and even the appearance of aging, we are not so sure that we want to face the inevitability of dying. Longevity and a fear of death have become near obsessions for the boomer generation.

Most of us do not feel the immediate, visceral impact of illness or death until we reach midlife, when parents and friends begin to die and/or when we ourselves are diagnosed with life-threatening illnesses. One woman suggested that boomers will not, in Dylan Thomas's words, go gently into that good night: "We will rage that we have not had enough sex or enough toys or enough heroic interventions. We are not a gracious bunch." A man in midlife said, "I hope we begin the transformation in a celebratory manner, leaving our loved ones loved and not abandoned."

Some older people seem better prepared. In an article "The Meaning of Aging" in the *Medical Post* (October 16, 2001), ninety-two-year-old psychiatrist Dr. Robert Weil writes, "We have to accept that life is terminal. That is the main complaint about old age – it's a short distance from death."

In her book *Necessary Losses* (1986), Judith Viorst suggests that denying death may make day-to-day life seem easier, but it will ultimately impoverish our lives. If we use so much energy now to fend off the fear and dread of death, we compromise our aliveness today and, paradoxically, limit the life we do have.

In our survey we asked, "What is your biggest worry about getting older and dying?" More than anything else, boomers fear aging and dying alone, without caring people around them. One woman responded, "My worst fear is dying alone without many or any family members to assist." People expressed fears of becoming ill, poor, and dependent on others, and of being cared for in an institution without family and friends around. They worry about dying too soon and leaving behind young children and unfinished family business. They worry about losing their partners and friends. "My mom and dad are in their late eighties," explains one woman. "The hardest thing for them is watching their friends and brothers and sisters die first. My mom says she is afraid to look at the obituary column in the paper because there is always someone she knows."

When asked "Where would you like to die?" the great majority said "at home" or "in my bed at home asleep." Some responses were more poetic: "with my wife by my side," "sitting in a lazy chair on a bluff overlooking the lake in early evening," "with the sun setting and a cool breeze wafting over my face." Said another, "It does not matter except *not* in a hospital."

### Changes in the Way We Will Die

Those who answered the Healthy Boomer Midlife Survey had a lot to say about how they believe the process of dying will differ for our generation compared with previous ones.

Midlife men and women expressed considerable apprehension about the double-edged sword of medical advances that may prolong life while robbing a dying person of a decent quality of life. Many cited their fear of being over-treated, with "tubes in every orifice," a predicament that makes the process of dying unnatural.

One man in his sixties said, "I am concerned about the tendency of medical professionals to try everything they can to keep people alive, even when the treatments have no chance of long-term success and cause suffering."

Other people worried that death would be longer and more drawn out. "As a result of medical interventions, the process of dying will be more protracted, institutional, and anonymous," said one woman. They spoke of their fear of pain and discomfort. "My family has bronchial problems," said one fifty-year-old man. "Everyone dies hard. Not being able to breathe scares me to death."

On the positive side, numerous people held out hopes that dying will be easier for the boomers than it was for their parents' generation. "I hope we will have more control than our parents did and will have given more conscious thought to our options," said one man. Some of these choices include medically assisted suicide, living wills, and more chances to die at home. Several suggested that better drugs will alleviate pain and suffering. "I feel lucky to be a Canadian and part of an affluent society," said one man. "I do believe there is much more care and attention available to us now."

## Midlife Orphan: When a Parent Dies

One of the most powerful experiences of midlife is the death of a parent. As Gail Sheehy writes in her book *New Passages: Mapping Your Life Across Time* (1995), "It throws you to the front of the generational train." You are it. There is no longer a parental buffer between you and the end. It can be a strange feeling to be someone without parents for the first time in your life, to be a "midlife orphan." We may feel bereft and lonely in surprising and disturbing ways, given that we've been earning a living, raising kids, and paying the mortgage for a few decades by now. One woman who had recently lost her father said, "I have always been so independent and really didn't see my dad that often, but when he was gone I felt strangely disoriented for a while. He'd always been there, and now he wasn't."

Tumultuous feelings from the past may arise, including unresolved conflicts and confusing, contradictory emotions of love, need, injustice, and anger. Journalist **Christie Blatchford**, in her column in the *National Post* (January 12, 2002), wrote a frank and unsentimental account of her mother's death. She began with "Everything they tell you about the death of a parent is true, only worse. It is always a surprise, no matter what."

When we talked with Christie, she said that, as she watched her mother slowly die, she would think, "I don't have kids; this could be me; who will look after me? It definitely brought me closer to my own death." She said that while she didn't want to die in an old-age home, "paying strangers to wipe my bum," she'd learned that in the end most of us choose life, whatever indignities this costs us. She noticed that her mother's mind would protect her from the reality of the worst invasive procedures. She simply didn't remember them and she would carry on as if everything was fine when she felt better. This gave her daughter some small comfort as she watched her mother's struggle.

Christie also spoke about how absolutely exhausted she herself felt. Not only was there the physical and emotional care of her mother, but the hours and hours she spent working the system, the long to-do list every day that never shrank. This included finding appropriate care when her mother's condition was continually changing, talking with doctors and social workers, as well as trying to carry on a work life and riding the roller coaster of emotions. Christie said, "None of the little stuff goes away just because you're bereft and hassled."

When we asked her how she kept herself going, she said she hadn't done a great job of it. While she knew that friends meant well when they said "take care of yourself," she said there just was no time to be good to herself. She remarked that most of the visitors on her mother's hospital ward seemed to be middle-aged women, whom she knew would have work and family responsibilities as well. "How the hell do they manage?" she asked. The most useful thing any friend could do was visit her mother for her. As Christie explained, "It gave me tremendous psychic relief, if I was out of town or held up, that a friend and not a paid stranger was there with her."

We asked what she might have done differently and she answered, "I did well; I did okay. I try not to think about what I could have done differently or better. I did my best. If I could have done anything differently, I would have touched her more. I did it as often as I could. Even with the yelling and anger, just being there is the key, just being there."

A forty-five-year-old woman in our survey described her experience with her dying mother this way: "She became emotionally distant and isolated. She was full of chemo. Her breast was removed. It was very difficult to watch this strong woman struggle with her disease. I felt depressed and angry. The hospital system was a nightmare. She died in the hospital at night, unconscious, with a morphine drip."

A fifty-four-year-old woman had quite a different experience. "My mother's death was rather beautiful. She was supported with good painkillers and lots of friends and family around her. Being with my mother's dead body was peaceful, but so 'not her.' I mean, she was no longer there. It was mystical."

### Looking after Each Other

Many boomers expressed concern about becoming burdens to their families when they got old and while dying. One man said, "I do not like the idea of medical advances extending my life beyond the point of enjoyment. If I am not enjoying life, my caregivers will probably resent caring for me. I like the idea of no heroics." Several people admitted they feared they would become burdens, because they might not be able to decide when it was time to die or to be allowed to die when they wanted to.

People expressed concern that family size has changed, and that our modern withdrawal from death makes family members less able to assist. "Perhaps we don't handle it as well as our forefathers," suggested one woman. "Family is less involved in the direct care of the dying than they used to be." One man said, "The sense of family responsibility to care for our elders is not nearly as strong as it used to be." Another simply pointed out that "many of us will be more alone, because families are so much smaller or in many cases, as with myself and my wife, there are no children."

The generation that banded together in new forms of cooperative living is now wondering if they can recreate that vision. Will we be able to create communities to help each other and how can that happen when we all become old?

One group of friends we spoke with is playing with the idea of developing a cooperative housing project on land one of the couples has purchased on the West Coast. "The idea is that we would pool our talents and help each other out. We have an accountant, an investor, a physician, a nurse, and a lot of other talented people in our group. We would build flexible housing, so that couples and friends who are alone could have independent housing, but there would also be communal space, such as a joint kitchen. People who wanted or needed help with cooking could do it together. And when we are all too old or sick, we will hire help."

Preparing for the Inevitable

Fifty-three-year-old **Brenda** and her two sons, **Dan** and **Michael**, talked with us about the recent loss of Robert, her husband and the boys' father. Brenda said, "When my husband was dying, I found the last few days very frustrating. It was incredible how Robert accepted one stage of his illness after the next. He was going to take any treatment as long as he had dignity and some quality of life. But at the end, the oncologist kept offering him more and more chemotherapy, even when we knew we were losing the fight. It seemed as if it was more for them than for Robert, as if the doctors had trouble accepting the defeat. Robert was very peaceful. He had prepared himself and both of our boys as well."

Dan said, "After the surgery we had hope, but I was not prepared for the chemotherapy and what followed. At the end, when my father was home before he died, I was away at university. It was hard to talk to Dad; he was so short of breath toward the end." Michael added, "I found it hard when he was home dying. It was hard to escape it. He was here all the time. There was no place to get away from it. I found it so hard to be optimistic."

When we asked Dan and Michael what helped them during this difficult time, Michael answered, "A friend of mine who had lost a parent as well was the best help. She felt the same way as I did and had the same experiences with relatives and friends." Michael also found that talking with a professional helped. He encouraged Michael to talk to his father, even if he couldn't talk back. "So, one day," said Michael, "I sat beside him and I talked."

Dan said that talking about the situation should not be forced. He said, "It may help some, but it was not for me. You have to get on with your life. I knew Dad would want me to go on."

Both recognized that the funeral was not held for them. "It was a lot of work and there was a lot of pressure on us. None of that was for us; it was all for the relatives." For Dan and Michael, because their father was suffering and because they knew he was going to die, death was "a relief and a release."

When we asked the brothers what their advice would be to friends who want to offer support, their suggestions were very practical:

- "It really helped when people just talked to us normally. It was such a relief when a family friend asked about my soccer team."

- "When you call, just leave a message. Ask if all is well and say 'You do not have to call back if you are okay.' Most of the time, you just don't feel like calling anybody back to answer the same questions over and over."
- "Just be there, with no expectations."
- "Drop off some food. Getting some fresh, warm food was always the best treat. After a long day of visiting the hospital and worrying about Dad, the last thing you want to worry about is food."

Dr. Lhotsky, who has worked with the dying in a chronic-care hospital, has observed that most people are not as prepared as Robert and his family were. Many are not as peaceful and accepting as Robert was, and most families are not as candid and open as Brenda, Dan, and Michael.

Dr. Lhotsky describes a more typical meeting of a medical team and family. "The team – nurses, social worker, and doctor – would sit in a meeting room with the close family members, going through a variety of scenarios to prepare for the time of death. We would discuss each scenario in detail. 'If your eighty-eight-year-old father with end-stage heart failure has a cardiac arrest, what would you like us to do? What if he gets pneumonia? How aggressive should our treatment be?' We would review all the criteria and options: when to give or not give intravenous fluids and when to use just 'comfort measures.' But when one of these situations arrived for real, the relatives and patients themselves would start to panic. Everybody would get very emotional. Very often, their well-thought-out plans would go out the window."

Maybe it is impossible to ever be completely ready, because each death, like each person, is unique. Or maybe we need to first become more comfortable and accepting of aging, illness, and dying as a normal stage at the end of life.

We asked **Patricia Daines**, R.N., M.N., a clinical nurse specialist in the Palliative Care Initiative at Sunnybrook and Women's College Health Sciences Centre in Toronto, Ontario, "Does it help us to prepare ourselves for the inevitable?" Her response confirms the dilemma we face when the medical establishment sees death as a failure rather than the end of the natural cycle of aging.

Pat says, "My first thought would be yes, it is better to prepare oneself. But on further reflection, I would say no. Logically, it should be easier to die if we prepare ourselves. But it is not. People used to die more naturally at home, but now, with our high-tech capacities and facilities, the goal has become to keep people alive. The medical establishment and patients themselves are always searching for something more. So one can be prepared, but often when things start to unravel, patients and families are confronted with too many choices."

"Doctors play a large role in the lives of the terminally ill," says **Mary Vachon**, R.N., Ph.D., and associate professor in the departments of Psychiatry and Public Health Sciences at the University of Toronto. "They are taught in medical school to cure people and to see death as a failure. Their education should also help them to deal with their own issues around death, but in all fairness, patients and their families have to be clear themselves about what they want.

"People are not interested in finding out about death ahead of time; they do not have the desire to reflect until they are personally touched by death. I spent thirty years dealing with patients with cancer, but everything changed when I had to deal with it myself. I have survived five years with lymphoma. I am now officially cured. I thought about death many times before the diagnosis, but more in the practical sense, such as having a living will. This totally changed when I was diagnosed. My journey was a spiritual and mystical one. From this personal experience, I now know, if you deal with death, you have more energy to live."

She describes how some people who meditate about dying come to a greater acceptance of death. But even they are afraid when the real threat of death arrives. Mary says, "In the book *Remarkable Recovery* [by Carlyle Hirshberg and Marc Barasch, 1995], investigators interviewed people and found several common denominators for spontaneous remissions of illnesses. They included strong relationships with others, spiritual beliefs, a sense of humor, good relationships with their doctors, participating in artistic endeavors, and maintaining a healthy diet.

"I always talk with my patients about healing as opposed to curing," Mary says. "I tell them that science and medicine may cure them, but it is understanding the meaning of illness that will help them to heal. Through illness, people may come to know themselves for the first time. They recognize not only who they genuinely are but also what really matters to them."

## Searching for "a Good Death"

Experts at the World Health Organization talk about "a good death." Under these circumstances, the dying person chooses the location of death and who will be with him or her. The patient and the family are well informed, their decisions are respected, and death is a peaceful experience. Compassionate care is available, suffering is minimized, and pain control is complete, both physical and spiritual. But what we see as "a good death" for one person may not be the same as it is for others.

As a palliative-care nurse, **Pat Daines** reflects on what professionals in the medical community would call a good death. "Some professionals like a quick death, others a more sedated and quiet exit. Yet we know that some patients would prefer to put up with discomfort, in order not to be too sedated. A person's death is as individual as his or her life. We need to respect people's rights. Those who like to have control until the end should have it. Sometimes we take away that control with drugs and technical interventions. I often wonder if it is our discomfort or theirs that we are treating.

"Who am I to say which death is good? Does it mean a death is bad if it is not peaceful enough for my taste? I may be uncomfortable with another person's choice, but that does not mean it is bad."

## Making Peace with Death

Spirituality plays a powerful role during dying. Friends and people in our survey who shared their experiences with dying relatives repeatedly suggested that having some form of spiritual faith helped the dying and those left behind.

One fifty-five-year-old man described the way his aunt died. "She was sick as a child, lost a lung to TB, and spent most of her life in poor health. She was deeply religious and never married. When she was ill she went to the hospital with her brothers, sisters, nieces, and nephews. We all went in and said our goodbyes. She felt bad for us, and as we prayed for her to hold on she would struggle to breathe. Finally, my uncle said, 'It is okay, Lois, it is time to go if you want.' A calmness came over her. She smiled, took a last breath, and was gone."

Another midlife man talked about his experience with his mother, who died five years earlier. "We talked. She knew she was going to die, and asked me to look after my brother. She believed in God, as I do. Even though there was a great sadness in me, I knew deep down she was going to a better place. I do not want to die, but I am not afraid of dying either. My mother taught me this."

Death is often the trigger for us to re-examine our spiritual beliefs, as this forty-five-year-old woman describes: "When my father died, I really had to face my vaguely defined thoughts about spirituality and afterlife. I was really quite confused about it. One day, however, I was out West skiing. It was a few months after his death. My friends and I decided to hike to a peak a short distance off with our skies and backpacks on our backs. I was immediately reminded of my dad and how he must have skied in his native Austria many years ago. As there were very few lifts at that time, skiing consisted of a very long hike up the mountain, followed by one extended run through untouched powder. All of a sudden, I felt him there with me. I knew he was there, experiencing and enjoying the hike with me. From then on, I felt easier. Somehow I knew he was still enjoying his beloved mountains, forest, and outdoor life."

Pat Daines talks about a woman she is seeing who is dying of a chronic end-stage illness: "She has such a shining spirit. She has taught me that, if people are able to get in touch with their inner selves, they will have an easier death. Her spiritual journey has taken her to a higher place and a deeper understanding of her reason for being. People may be bound by pain and physical limitations and yet be spiritually free. This gives their death meaning."

## The Final Lesson

"We all live with the possibility of death, but the dying live with the probability," says Elisabeth Kübler-Ross, an expert on death and dying (in *Two Experts on Death and Dying Teach Us About the Mysteries of Life and Living*, 2000). She goes on to say that "we all have lessons to learn during this time called life; this is especially apparent when working with the dying. The dying learn a great deal at the end of life, usually when it is too late to apply it." Can we learn the lessons of dying while we are alive and healthy?

The knowledge that we will die can heighten and fine-tune our sense of the moment. We heard over and over again how people who are confronted with a terminal illness suddenly change. They begin to live every moment more fully, with a new sense of purpose and peace.

"People who've become aware of their mortality find that they've gained the freedom to live," writes Bernie Segal in his essay "Love: The Work of Soul," in the *Handbook for the Soul* by Richard Carlson and Benjamin Shield (1996). As one woman said, "The first thing I did after I was diagnosed with cancer was to get rid of my 'draining' friends and acquaintances. I knew I needed to be spending time with people who were nurturing, not draining, me."

In her book *My Grandfather's Blessings* (2000), author Rachel Naomi Remen writes about the meaning of life. "Finding meaning does not require us to live differently; it requires us to see life differently." Our survey respondents told us how they learned the lessons of death and ultimately to see life differently by being with loved ones as they die. One fifty-year-old man described how a friend managed her death. "She arranged for her own support group, which met regularly for fellowship and a discussion about how each of us felt as she went through the dying process over a one-year period. Being with someone at the terminal stage of life helped me examine my own feelings about dying."

### Leaving a Legacy

For many people, leaving a legacy is also an important way by which they can come to terms with letting go of life. **Kate Carmichael** was one of those people. For those who don't live in Halifax, Carmichael was probably best known through her outspoken discussions with Shelagh Rogers on CBC Radio's *This Morning* show. Kate spoke bluntly and fearlessly about her battle with leukemia and about her feelings about dying. She compared her fear of dying to the fear of giving birth. She said that you wonder how it will happen, but you become mellower as you get closer to it, realizing that hundreds of thousands have gone before you. Kate had been the executive director of the Downtown Halifax Business Commission since 1996, and was credited with a major revitalization of the downtown area. She was also known as the "godmother of the craft movement," conceiving and organizing the first large craft market in Nova Scotia, twenty-five years ago. At her memorial service, friends joked that she had left a to-do list for them to carry on the work she began. One fellow councilor said, "Her enduring legacy will continue to burn brightly." Kate was fifty-one when she died on October 17, 2001.

## From the Research
### *Seven Factors That Predict Healthy Aging*
The landmark Harvard Study of Adult Development has followed three cohorts of men and women since 1938 in an effort to find the key factors that predict health and happiness in old age. The study has shown that at age fifty, the following factors are the best predictors of good physical and psychosocial health at age seventy:

1. no heavy smoking
2. good coping skills (emotional maturity) and a wide social support network
3. no alcohol abuse (defined as having alcohol-related problems with one's spouse, family, employer, law, or own health)
4. a healthy weight
5. stable marriage/relationship
6. some exercise
7. more than twelve years of education

Source: Vaillant, George E. *Aging Well: Surprising Guideposts to a Happier Life from the Landmark Harvard Study of Adult Development*, 2002.

### *Defining a "Good Death" in a Nursing Home*
One in four Americans who reaches the age of sixty-five will die in a nursing home, yet little research exists to define the end-of-life care needs of this segment of the population. In focus groups with seventy-seven participants, nursing-home residents cited lack of training, insufficient resources, and inflexible regulations as important barriers to high-quality care of the dying in nursing homes. Three major themes emerged to define a good death in a nursing home:

- highly individualized care based on a continuity of relationships with familiar caregivers;

- effective teamwork by staff, physicians, and family; and
- comprehensive planning that addresses prognosis, emotional preparation, and the appropriate use of medical treatments.

Source: Hanson, L. C., M. Henderson, and M. Menon. "As Individual as Death Itself: A Focus Group Study of Terminal Care in Nursing Homes," *Journal of Palliative Medicine*, Vol. 5, No. 1 (2002): 117–25.

## On the Lighter Side

*How Old Is Grandpa?*

One evening, a boy was talking with his grandfather about current events. He asked the older man what he thought about the shootings at schools, the computer age, and things in general.

The granddad replied, "Well, let me think a minute. I was born before television, penicillin, polio shots, frozen foods, Xerox, contact lenses, Frisbees, and the Pill. There were no radar, credit cards, laser beams, or ballpoint pens. Man had not invented pantyhose, air conditioners, dishwashers, clothes dryers, and the clothes were hung out to dry in the fresh air. Man had not yet walked on the moon.

"Pizza Hut and McDonald's were unheard of. There were five-and-ten-cent stores where you could actually buy things for five and ten cents. Ice-cream cones, phone calls, rides on a streetcar, and a Pepsi all cost a nickel. If you didn't want to splurge, you could spend your nickel on enough stamps to mail one letter and two postcards. You could buy a new Chevy Coupe for $600, but who could afford one? Too bad, because gas was 11 cents a gallon.

"My childhood was before gay rights, computer-dating, dual careers, daycare centers, and group therapy. Your grandmother and I got married first – and then lived together. Having a meaningful relationship meant getting along with your cousins. 'Time sharing' meant spending time with the family together in the evenings.

"In my day, 'grass' was mowed, 'coke' was a cold drink, 'pot' was something your mother cooked in, 'chip' meant a piece of wood, 'hardware' was found in a hardware store, and 'software' wasn't even a word.

"And how old do you think I am?"

This man would be only fifty-eight years old!

## Questions to Reflect On

Relationships with people who are dying, as well as a conscious acceptance of our own aging and mortality, can help us avoid "simply having visited the world." Instead, we hope that this awareness will help us embrace the world today with more wonder and amazement.

1. For you, what are three things that are positive about aging?
2. Imagine that you are told that you have only five months to live. What is one thing you would change or do now that you always wanted to do?
3. What do you need to do to feel you've really been "here" in this life?
4. What message would you like to see on your grave marker?

CHAPTER THIRTEEN

# *The Soul Seekers*

And almost everyone when age,
Disease, or sorrows strike him,
Inclines to think there is a God,
Or something very like Him.

> – Arthur Hugh Clough, *Dipsychus,* 1862

Boomers are on a quest. We are following the ancient pilgrims' route to Santiago de Compostela in Spain; we're walking the labyrinth at Chartres Cathedral; we're going on retreats instead of on holidays. We're meditating, praying, studying the Koran, the Bible, and the Kabbalah, going to sweat lodges, and practicing yoga, tai chi, and ji gong like never before. We are looking for meaning and connection, something to help us keep the materialistic strivings of our generation in perspective. For some, the search is precipitated by a personal brush with death or the heart attack of a midlife neighbor who was just about to "slow down and smell the roses." For others, it is a vague, uneasy feeling that something is missing, that there must be more to existence than just this physical plane. In this chapter we explore what our survey respondents, interview subjects, and other experts have to say about spirituality in midlife. We remain amazed at the richness and commitment we heard in their stories and very grateful to those who shared their experiences with us – and you, the reader.

### The Meaning of Spirituality

While researching *The Healthy Boomer,* we were repeatedly asked why we had not included questions about spirituality in our first questionnaire. This was important to so many people we talked with that eventually we included a chapter specifically on spiritual well-being. Since then, much has been written about the boomers' search for answers, ranging from stories of individual spiritual odysseys to guides to spiritual retreats and handbooks of personally chosen prayers. In the aftermath of September 11, 2001, concerns about the meaning of life and spiritual values seem even more important.

In the Healthy Boomer Midlife Survey, we posed the question "What does spirituality mean to you?" To most of those who responded, it meant a sense of connection to some higher power and a belief in something greater than themselves. Here are some of their answers:

- "Spirituality nourishes me and gives me a perspective for living a meaningful life."
- "I have a strong belief in being part of a greater plan."
- "It is the best part of us all – pure golden energy which can propel me into greatness."
- "It is simply inner peace."
- "Being spiritual helps me cope with life and its challenges, and to stay balanced all around."
- "It connects me with both the human race and an ultimate power, which is indescribable and unexplained."
- "Spirituality enables me to remind myself what the important things are in life. It helps me keep everyday stress in perspective."

Some 45 per cent of respondents to the survey stated that spirituality has always been important to them. Many of these boomers have consistently practiced the faiths of their childhoods. About one-quarter (26%) had returned to the faiths of their childhoods. Some 39 per cent had explored new directions.

For many, spirituality is a personal matter that has little to do with the organized religion in which they were raised. One fifty-year-old woman spoke vehemently of "not liking and not trusting organized religion." One man said, "Organized religion does not have a large place in my vision of spirituality." Yet some spoke of a comforting return to a church, synagogue, or mosque after a long hiatus:

- "It used to be a struggle to go to church. Recently, I have found it a place of refuge, quiet reflection, and peace. A place of solitude.

When I am there, I visit places in my soul that take away the confusion and negative emotions that would otherwise overwhelm me. I
leave feeling light and refreshed."

- "The church service helps me focus on others instead of myself. It
  reminds me of what is important in life and to enjoy each moment.
  It reminds me to give in all ways without expectation of return,
  because it is the giving that makes one happy."

Some still doubt. A fifty-six-year-old man told us, "I am not sure. I struggle
with the Christian concepts of God and spirituality, at least God in the
context of my own personal life. Although I am a churchgoer and embrace
a Christian philosophical view, I don't have a strong spiritual life and I am
somewhat cynical now about those who say they do."

Other boomers have fashioned their own forms of spirituality from the
philosophies and practices of different faiths and from humanistic psy-
chology and New Age thinking. Gone are the days when people would
simply say they were Catholic or Jewish or Protestant. Many boomers
interested in spiritual seeking have complex, eclectic approaches. One
woman wrote, "Spirit is a place I go to. I would love to spend some more
time exploring native spiritual beliefs. I also plan to study Buddhism more,
as this is fascinating to me." Another described her sense of spirituality as
"a belief in a life hereafter, in reincarnation, that our souls choose to learn
particular lessons and work through accumulated Karma from previous
lives on earth." Another said spirituality is "that part of us that goes beyond
the hardware and software of our existence, that connects us to the past and
the future, the collective unconscious that Jung referred to." Others spoke
of spirituality from a humanistic perspective. "What a question!" wrote a
fifty-five-year-old woman raised in the Jewish faith. She went on, "Okay,
here goes. It means living with a sense of awe, wonder, blessing, gratitude,
adventure, joy, harmony, love, humor, connectedness, intimacy, beauty,
and the rhythms of music and dance."

The breadth of these answers illustrates this generation's belief in their
right and ability to create a form of spirituality unique to themselves. As
with many other aspects of their lives, boomers are not comfortable with
following in the steps of those who have gone before. Their rebellion
against authority extends to organized religions. While this is not true for

all of this age group, the dwindling numbers in many mainstream churches and synagogues seem to support this general premise.

### SOME HIGHLIGHTS FROM THE HEALTHY BOOMER MIDLIFE SURVEY

| *How important is spirituality to you at present?* | |
| --- | --- |
| It has always been important. | 45% |
| It has become increasingly important. | 30% |
| It has become less important. | 10% |
| It has never been important. | 15% |

| *If it is important to you, have you . . . ?* | |
| --- | --- |
| Returned to the faith of your childhood | 26% |
| Explored new directions | 40% |
| Not applicable | 21% |
| Other | 13% |

### The Importance of Spirituality

Almost one-third of the boomers who answered our survey said that spirituality has become increasingly important to them in midlife. When we asked them to tell us a story about the importance of spirituality right now, the replies were rich and varied:

- "In times of sadness or loss or of great happiness and thankfulness, I am comforted and renewed by nature, by music, and by people. I also take great comfort in my religion. Although I don't practice it all the time formally, it is part of me and I seem to carry it with me all the time."
- "Spirituality is my compass. I always check in with my soul to find the best direction for me. My inner spiritual voice guides me through life's obstacles and helps me get to the other side."
- "This is a story about awareness and elevated consciousness that happens to me nearly every day. I walk with my dog down by the ocean. I throw a few sticks, and I am exhilarated with her zest for

play. She explores in the water and I do a few stretches. If it is dark, I notice the pattern of sand left on the kelp from my dog's churning feet in the spray of phosphorescent light. Slowly my thoughts leave my inner self. Then, I find myself on the beach again, really feeling the wind in my face, seeing the long heave of the waves. Just being alive."

• "Without my connection to spirit, my life would be empty and morose. I find my happiness and my very sustenance in my spirit. It gives me everything I need and affords me enormous peace."

Several people noted that spirituality reminds them of the importance of forgiveness. One woman said, "When I feel resentful or angry toward someone, I feel robbed of the stillness that is central to a spiritual life. Forgiveness is a gift we need to give to ourselves as well as to others." Other boomers spoke of being brought to greater spiritual awareness through dealing with personal illness and physical limitations, or the death of a family member or friend.

• "When I was diagnosed with prostate cancer, I had a great moment of enlightenment in the car, when I started to cry. I explained to my wife that I needed something to help me get through this experience. The word 'universe' popped into my head. There was an immediate sense that I was part of everything and everything was part of me. This feeling was powerful. It filled my body. I could feel the power that was out there and in myself to keep me well. I calmed down and stopped crying. I remember thinking, if anything is going to help, this was it."

• "My physical body is something of a wreck. I wake up every morning in pain. My knees and hips ache much of the time. I often have debilitating headaches. I can't walk far without getting out of breath and can't walk at all in cold weather without precipitating an asthmatic attack. When I go into the city or even walk on the beautiful nearby beach, I often get a cold or sore throat. In short, I have serious physical limitations. That being said, I still have a rich and full life, brimming with beauty, intimacy, curiosity about new things, rejoicing and working for good causes. My life is grounded in the spiritual plane."

• "I believe my mother is still looking after me and my family. I visit her grave regularly. If I am having a bad day, I pray to her and something good always happens."

## Religious Vocations in Midlife

Paradoxically, while there has been a decrease in the number of boomers belonging to churches and synagogues, there has been an increase in the number of boomers turning to religion as a second career. In Canada, an astonishing 96 per cent of Anglican clergywomen have had previous careers and are in "a second vocation." Twenty-five years ago, women made up only 1 per cent of the Anglican clergy; today the figure is closer to 25 per cent.

On October 19, 2001, even the *Wall Street Journal* documented the increase in religious vocations for boomers, reporting that in 1999 nearly one-quarter of the seminary graduates in North America were over age fifty. Many were pursuing a second career after succeeding in earlier careers as varied as airline pilot, pig farmer, physicist, police officer, chartered accountant, and cowboy. Now, many faith institutions actively recruit older candidates, citing the valuable professional skills and life experience they bring to their jobs. Those who turn to these second careers describe themselves as feeling deeply rewarded by helping others. Perhaps equally satisfying for them is the connection between their ministry work and the development of their own souls.

When she was in her early forties, **Joan** left her job as a CBC television producer and eventually became a fully ordained Zen Buddhist monk. She explains, "Traditional religion was never relevant to me; it had too many conflicting stories. I was searching for what was true of this life." She went to Africa to work in development broadcasting in remote areas. While she was there, she continued her lifelong search for something that had meaning to her. She investigated several different Eastern practices, including transcendental meditation. But Zen Buddhism fascinated her the most. "The aesthetics, the history, and the practice of Zen made undeniable experiential sense to me," she says. Back in Ottawa, she read an article about the practice of Zen at a local center. When she called, the Zen Master invited her to meet with him at 5:30 the next morning. "I have never looked back. I have been practicing and studying with him since 1988. In May of 2001,

I received transmission as his Dharma heir." Joan now lives in a Zen Buddhist monastery full-time. Since her ordination, she has introduced hundreds of people to the practice of mindfulness and mind-body education at Zen workshops throughout North America and Europe. "I am content," she says, "and my work is gratifying. I have no regrets. Each moment is a joy practicing this life that lives as all of us."

### Spirituality and Western Medicine

While spirituality has always played a central role in traditional indigenous healing, it has not been considered relevant to the scientific methods of western medicine until fairly recently. However, in the last five to ten years, a growing number of research papers have cited the powerful, positive influence of prayer and meditation. A medical colleague said she was shocked to see an article in the October 9, 2001, *Medical Post* entitled "God's Place in Medicine." As she put it, "Even a few years ago we would never have seen an article like this." The piece elicited responses that ranged from an enthusiastic acknowledgment of the need for prayer shared by physician and patient to shocked reactions that there is no place in medicine for either politics or religion.

**Dr. Glenn Jones**, a radiation oncologist at the Hamilton Regional Cancer Centre, has developed a research program that studies the association between spirituality and the ways people make treatment decisions and cope with cancer. When we interviewed him, Dr. Jones explained that he is developing and testing a reliable and valid way to measure core health-related spirituality and to determine a connection between spirituality, the management or treatment chosen, and a patient's cancer prognosis. This field of research as a whole is still in its infancy, particularly in cancer management.

He and his colleagues have developed a questionnaire that surveys patients in fifteen different areas of spirituality. The questionnaire includes four different categories of spirituality that patients have identified as most important to them during their cancer experiences: coping and hoping, dealing with loss, understanding purpose and meaning, and developing a greater awareness of any supernatural side to reality. The last category refers to transcendence, powers, and deities on the one hand, and personal spiritual resources and function on the other hand. Dr. Jones and colleagues are administering the questionnaires and conducting interviews to evaluate how personal spirituality influences decisions and experiences. "In the next two years we hope to have developed strong measures that will move the field forward in a significant manner," he says, "so that we may start measuring the effects of interventions like meditation and chemo-radiation in patient populations."

"One way to look at spirituality," says Dr. Jones, "is to see it as the C.E.O. of the human system which brings together the body, mind, and emotions and seeks to create a harmony among them. Disease may be the dishar-mony or dysfunction in any of these four aspects of our being." He suggests that modern medicine has focused a lot of research at the level of the single cell in the past few decades, and with great success. Now a lot of research is being done on the human genome, looking for genetic causes of disease at the very center of the cell. But to truly understand disease, medicine must also look at larger types of organization and not just that within a single cell. Humans are whole persons, each an interconnected entity that includes spirituality. Dr. Jones and his colleagues believe that this perspec-tive provides a vital framework that can help explain why therapies as varied as sound waves, meditation, acupuncture, prayer, deep breathing, and therapeutic touch can influence the development and course of a disease such as cancer.

At age thirty-nine, **Janet** was diagnosed with malignant melanoma. Three years later, the cancer had spread. She was told that she had six months to live. Nine months of chemotherapy treatments made her extremely sick. "It was a living hell," she said. "There was no relief from the vomiting."

Janet describes how a stranger came to her house one day, accompanied by his four-year-old son. They had been praying in a church nearby, and sensed that she needed help. "He told me that I would find the strength to get better, that I would pull through this," says Janet. "I do not know how he knew, but it was not important. He blessed our house and left."

She told us that, from that point on, she started to feel stronger. She found help in therapeutic touch and was further encouraged by a healer. As she was getting stronger, she started to exercise and eat well. She got involved in Wellspring, a support program for cancer patients. For now, all of her lesions are gone except for one small spot on her liver that is not growing.

"I have become very strong spiritually during this illness," says Janet. "I know I can do anything now. I have no fear. I believe that, after what I have been through, God is not going to take away my life. Spirituality is part of my daily life now. I get up every morning and open my arms as wide as I can to accept the good energy into my body and move away the bad energy. I pray and thank God for each day. Occasionally, I wonder if people will believe that all this is possible. But then I realize it does not matter. This is my life and I want to live it the best I can!"

### Spirituality and the Workplace

If spirituality and western medicine have had an uneasy relationship, spirituality and the business world have seemed hopelessly incompatible. But, slowly, this too is beginning to change. In 1994, poet David Whyte published a bestselling book, *The Heart Aroused: Poetry and the Preservation of the Soul in Corporate America*. The book is based on his own experience in working with executives of Fortune 500 companies through poetry and story in order to "bring the insights of the poetic imagination out of the garret and into the board rooms and factory floors of America." Whyte describes how male executives approaching fifty years of age often feel discontent and long for something beyond the daily grind. He says that, in midlife, we may find "a corpse across our doorway" that on closer examination bears an uncanny resemblance to our lost dreams and "former intuitions for a possible life." With a conscious effort to acknowledge this, the road of midlife can be a "newer and more profound path to meaningful work." He adds that "preserving the soul means that we come out of hiding at last and bring more of ourselves into the workplace."

In 2001, Ann Coombs, a business consultant, published *The Living Workplace: Soul, Spirit and Success in the 21st Century*. In this Canadian bestseller, she challenges corporations to attend to the spiritual needs of their people – their most valuable resource. She conducts workshops to help companies create spiritually friendly environments that encourage employees to bring all of their talents – of body, mind, heart, and soul – to work.

What is perhaps so startling is not that these books were written but that they have generated an enormously positive response. This may indicate that the burden of keeping our work separate from what has deep meaning for us has become simply too much to bear. In David Whyte's most recent book, *Crossing the Unknown Sea: Work as a Pilgrimage of Identity* (2001), he makes a strong case for work's being a means of knowing our true nature, rather than an obstacle to it. He cites the need for "new conversations in the workplace," where both the needs of the organization and the needs of the individual for vitality, imagination, and soulfulness can stand a better chance of being realized.

### Understanding the Spiritual Quest

So what is the boomers' spiritual quest all about? We asked philosopher and writer, **Peter Emberley**, for his thoughts about this. Peter wrote *Divine Hunger: Canadians on a Spiritual Walkabout* (2002), which is based on a study of the baby boomers' search for spiritual meaning. In researching the book, he visited a number of retreat centers and monasteries. He participated in a Sioux sweat lodge, attended a New Age Spiritfest, went to the Jesus Seminar meetings, and visited Swami Shyam's International Meditation Institute (IMI) in Kullu, India.

In a recent conversation with us, Peter spoke of the complex and sometimes confusing nature of the boomers' spiritual journey. There are many contradictions. On the one hand, people in this stage of their lives feel a deep spiritual longing and questioning. On the other hand, many have a rebellious adolescent disdain for the past and the undeniable narcissism of the Big Generation – the belief that "it must be important because I'm doing it." Boomers often express a wish for community and connection, yet many have rejected the old forms of religion, which offered many previous generations the very sense of comfort and community that boomers now seek. There is an eclecticism rich in creative experimentation, but lacking in a rigorous self-discipline that has long been considered an essential part of spiritual growth.

Many men and women in our survey, as well as many people with whom Peter spoke, made a sharp distinction between being spiritual and being religious, as if the two are somehow incompatible. In the boomers' attempt to define themselves as different from all who have gone before, they may have inadvertently thrown the proverbial baby out with the bath water. Many boomers feel the lack of a structure and form in which to act on this spiritual yearning while ignoring the fact that they have rejected the structure that more traditional religions provide. The Reverend Lynn Artress explained this distinction in her 1995 book, *Walking a Sacred Path*: "We have confused religion with spirituality, the container with the process. Religion is the outward form, the container, specifically the liturgy and all the acts of worship. Spirituality is the inward activity of growth and maturation that happens in each of us."

Rejecting established religious forms has increased many boomers' spiritual awareness and insight. It has also left some adrift and bereft, with no community of worship, no teachings to follow and pass on to their children, and only vague longings for something more. Peter Emberley points out that others seem to have replaced going to church with an almost ritualized attendance at spiritual-growth seminars. Still others, such as those living at Swami Shyam's institute, who criticized the dogmatic, authoritarian structure of western religion, have found solace and belonging in the hierarchy of eastern religions, based on strict relations between the master and the disciple. Swami Shyam is a powerful authority figure who, Peter says, "sometimes functions as a challenging psychotherapist, a wise friend, or a benevolent parent." He notes that there is an element of the Peter Pan syndrome in the boomers' wish to find a protected world of unconditional love, safely away from the disappointments and limitations of the outside world. "Our problem is that we can't find a comfortable middle ground," he concludes.

"Many boomers have fashioned their own unique fusion faith," Peter explains, "with a little of this and a little of that." Because of this diversity, you might meet a Jewish Buddhist on silent retreat in Cape Breton or a United Church yoga practitioner at a Goddess retreat in Moose Jaw. The once unheard-of has become the ordinary.

**June Rogers**, a writer and health editor, described what spirituality means to her and how her husband's spiritual quest affected their son's decision about a coming-of-age ritual.

She remembers always knowing there was something more – "a deep knowledge," she calls it, "of something beyond myself." June was raised Roman Catholic, but was turned off by the church's dogma and authoritarian teachings. When we asked how she keeps a sense of the spiritual alive in daily life, she said that she focuses on "things that have meaning." This might mean compassionately listening to the fears of a friend who has just found a lump in her breast or helping a ninety-year-old neighbor get out of a funk after a recent fall. For June, spirituality is about "connecting deeply with another's soul." She also finds spiritual renewal in her community theater where, through singing, dancing, and acting, she feels "inspired and connected with the universe."

Her husband was raised in an orthodox Jewish home. She said he has always been searching, but became more active in his spiritual quest following the death of his father. Together, they attended a humanistic secular Jewish group for a number of years, which provided their son with a connection to his Jewish heritage. Interestingly, their son had the option of having a coming-of-age ritual within this secular group or a more traditional bar mitzvah. He chose the latter.

When asked about the effect midlife had on her spiritual sense, June replied, "It is deeper than it was. That sense of connectedness has never gone away. I don't know if there's a heaven or hell, or what will happen when I die, but it's okay not to know. I'll find out when I get there."

Is the boomers' spiritual questing just another example of self-absorption and self-indulgence? Peter says, "Despite all of the contradictions, we boomers deeply long for something authentic, and this longing is very genuine. Now [in midlife], many are experiencing the truth of the scripture, 'What is a man profited, if he shall gain the whole world, and lose his own soul?'"

We asked Peter what is driving the boomers' spiritual search. He said it was a combination of factors, including an increased awareness that life on earth is temporary and the fact that we are increasingly confronted with our own mortality in midlife. We also share a sincere desire to give our children some spiritual sense of life. He called our eclectic approach to our children's spiritual education "the spiritual equivalent of home schooling." As always, it seems that we choose what fits and what pleases us, without always reckoning with the loss of self-discipline and loss of connection and generosity to others that may result.

**Lucinda Vardey**, a former businesswoman, is now an author, yoga teacher, and pilgrimage leader. She and three other midlife women created The Catherine Collective to bring more of the language of the feminine into religious and spiritual discourse. The collective is named after St. Catherine of Siena. In an interview, Lucinda said how important it is to contemplate through meditation, but also to participate in a living spirituality of love in action. For Catherine Collective members, this means practicing the feminine way of "giving, receiving, and circulating" resources, be they money, goods, ideas, or prayer. Lucinda describes the collective's work as "putting love into action by promoting and practicing generosity and trying to make things and people better." The collective is currently raising money for a women's clinic in Afghanistan. Lucinda told us that 100 per cent of what is received goes immediately into this project and other help for women in need. She remarked that quite a few people have come into the collective feeling so depleted that they believe they have nothing to give. She says, "We have found repeatedly that, when the giving is experienced as giving to God, people have a surprising experience of replenishment." She noted that perhaps our generation's chronic feeling of "running on empty" is because we lack a spiritual dimension in our giving.

### From the Research
#### Religion and Longevity
In a study of some 126,000 people, scientists at the National Institute for Healthcare Research in the United States found that people who were more involved in their religions – for example, attending worship services frequently or spending spare time in religious activities – were almost 30 per cent more likely to live longer than those who were less involved.
Source: "Spiritual Matters, Earthly Benefits," *Tufts University Health & Nutrition Letter* (August 2001).

#### Spirituality and Earthly Benefits
In a study with participants in Dean Ornish's Lifestyle Heart Trial, spirituality scores were significantly related with the degree of progression or regression of coronary-artery obstruction over a four-year period. People with the lowest scores in spiritual well-being showed the greatest progression of coronary obstruction; those with the highest scores showed the most regression. In another study conducted by Duke University,

devout patients recovering from surgery spent an average of eleven days in hospital compared with non-religious patients who spent an average of twenty-five days!

Source: Morris, E. L. "The Relationship of Spirituality to Coronary Artery Disease." Franklin, North Carolina: Franklin Cardiac Rehabilitation Program, 2000.

## On the Lighter Side
*Church Bloopers*
The following are alleged to have appeared in church bulletins:

1. The Low Self-Esteem Support Group will meet Thursday at 7 p.m. Please use the back door.
2. The pastor will preach his farewell message, after which the choir will sing, "Break Forth into Joy."
3. A songfest was hell at the Methodist church Wednesday.
4. Remember in prayer the many who are sick of our church and community.
5. The eighth-graders will be presenting Shakespeare's *Hamlet* in the Church basement Friday at 7 p.m. The Congregation is invited to attend this tragedy.
6. Don't let worry kill you, let the church help.
7. For those of you who have children and don't know it, we have a nursery downstairs.
8. This being Easter Sunday, we will ask Mrs. Lewis to come forward and lay an egg on the altar.
9. Eight new choir robes are currently needed, due to the addition of several new members and to the deterioration of some older ones.

## Questions to Reflect On
1. Do you feel a longing for more spirituality in your life? If yes, identify the kind of things that nourish the sense of the spiritual in your day-to-day life (for example, listening to Beethoven, a nature walk, attending a faith service, praying, reading the Bible or a book of uplifting poetry). How can you incorporate these activities into your daily and weekly schedule?

2. If you are already a member of a faith community, what is one small thing you can do now to deepen your commitment and your connections to that community? As a reflection of your faith, how can you reach out and give to your broader community in a manageable, practical way?

3. How does your spirituality influence the ways you view your work? What one small thing could you do at work to contribute to a more spiritually friendly environment for everyone?

4. Do you believe that healing the spirit and healing the body go hand in hand? What small changes could you make to your spiritual outlook now that would improve your health and sense of well-being?

5. Do you want to explore new spiritual practices and beliefs? If yes, what is one small step you can take now to do so?

# CONCLUSION

# *One Year from Now*

In her poem "The Summer Day" (*New and Selected Poems*, 1992), Mary Oliver speaks eloquently about the opportunities for reflection and refocusing that midlife offers us:

Who made the world?
Who made the swan, and the black bear?
Who made the grasshopper?
This grasshopper, I mean –
the one who has flung herself out of the grass,
the one who is eating sugar out of my hand,
who is moving her jaws back and forth instead of up and down –
who is gazing around with her enormous and complicated eyes.
Now she lifts her pale forearms and thoroughly washes her face.
Now she snaps her wings open, and floats away.
I don't know exactly what a prayer is.
I do know how to pay attention, how to fall down
into the grass, how to kneel down in the grass,
how to be idle and blessed, how to stroll through the fields,
which is what I have been doing all day.
Tell me, what else should I have done?
Doesn't everything die at last, and too soon?
Tell me, what is it you plan to do
With your one wild and precious life?

Again and again, the people we spoke with told us they want to reclaim some of the joy and laughter and "wildness" they had lost in the serious business of adulthood. They told us that they want a better balance of work, play, and rest, time to meditate and time for art and music. They want to "just roll with the punches," to be more outgoing and more loving, to achieve serenity and build more long-lasting friendships. They want to know again how to "fall down in the grass" and "be idle" and feel "blessed" with what they have.

In midlife, we can no longer take our precious lives for granted. This period in our lives is a time of change, whether we want it to be or not. For so many of those we spoke with, a confrontation with a serious illness or the death of a friend became the wake-up call to them to finally begin to care for ourselves. As the poet reminds us, "Doesn't everything die at last, and too soon?"

We asked participants in the 2001 Healthy Boomer Midlife Survey, "If there were one thing you could change in your health during the coming year, what would it be?" Responses ran a full range of possibilities in the physical, spiritual, emotional, and social realms, from lowering cholesterol levels, becoming more mentally alert, and overcoming depression, to building more friendships and – we quote – "becoming spiritually connected to more than a chocolate!"

Their stories and observations echoed what we know about change. It is not easy, but it can be accomplished. It requires both a vision of where you'd like to be and the willingness and perseverance to take many small steps to get there. Those who take time to formulate a clear picture of the change, prepare for it thoughtfully, and take measured, consecutive steps towards it are more likely to succeed. Those who garner support from friends, family, community, and the environment are more likely to maintain those changes.

### What One Change Would You Like to Make This Year?

We did the following exercise together to help each of us develop a plan for one change we ourselves would like to make in the next year. We found it helpful. We hope you will, too.

This exercise asks you to visualize yourself one year from now, after you have successfully made one change that is important to you, and then write down exactly what you did to make it happen.

Doing this exercise can help us open our thinking and get out of the places where we usually become stuck. When we look at a specific change from the vantage point of its already having been achieved, we often find it easier to recognize that our perceived barriers to change may not be so insurmountable after all.

You can work on this exercise alone or with a friend. The friend's job is to listen and pose encouraging questions to help you create a detailed picture of your change and of the steps you took to make it happen.

As you go through the exercise, continue to think and speak about this change as if it has already been made. Be as specific and as honest with yourself as you can.

1.  Set aside a quiet time and place where you can reflect alone or with a good friend. Have a piece of paper and a pen nearby. Take a few minutes to relax and release tension by breathing deeply.

2.  Imagine that you are sitting in this spot one year from today, feeling proud and happy that you have accomplished one specific change that you set in motion during the last twelve months. Breathe deeply into this good and satisfied feeling.
    What was the change you made? Be detailed and very precise. It could be anything from losing ten pounds to going on weekly dates with your partner for a dinner and talk.

3.  Now, cast your thoughts back to the steps you took to reach that change.
    Ask yourself these questions:
    *   Why did you decide – finally – to make the change this time?
    *   How was this time different from the previous times you've thought about this change or tried to carry it out?
    *   What did you do to carefully prepare for success before you took action?
    *   What were all of the steps you took to achieve this change?
    *   Where did you run into roadblocks?
    *   How did you find a way around these roadblocks?
    *   What kind of support did you learn you needed?
    *   Who did you ask to give you that support?
    *   How did you reward yourself and reinforce the change?
    *   Having put this change firmly in place, how will you maintain it?

4. When you have thought this through, write down all the steps in detail.

5. Choose a starting date for your action plan and begin your preparation activities.

6. Remember that many people find it much harder to maintain a change than to start on one because they have not prepared sufficiently for lasting change. Don't despair if you slide back. Analyze what you have learned, revise your goal, and start again. Then use what you have learned to prepare yourself better the next time.

**Over to You Now**

As we collected the stories for this book, we were continually touched by the honesty, humor, wit, and wisdom that our midlife respondents shared with us. Their experiences inspired us to make changes in our own lives. Now it is your turn.

# A FINAL WORD

We would be happy to receive your comments about this book and to hear about your experiences in midlife. Please contact us at:

The Toronto Midlife Health Institute
90 Eglinton Avenue East, Suite 402
Toronto, Ontario
Canada
M 4 P 2 Y 3
Web: www.healthyboomer.com